Uveitis

C. Stephen Foster
Stephen D. Anesi • Peter Y. Chang
Editors

Uveitis

A Quick Guide to Essential Diagnosis

Springer

Editors
C. Stephen Foster, MD, FACS, FACR
Massachusetts Eye Research and Surgery Institution
Ocular Immunology and Uveitis Foundation
Waltham, MA
USA

Stephen D. Anesi, MD, FACS
Massachusetts Eye Research and Surgery Institution
Ocular Immunology and Uveitis Foundation
Waltham, MA
USA

Peter Y. Chang, MD
Massachusetts Eye Research and Surgery Institution
Ocular Immunology and Uveitis Foundation
Waltham, MA
USA

ISBN 978-3-030-52973-4 ISBN 978-3-030-52974-1 (eBook)
https://doi.org/10.1007/978-3-030-52974-1

This Springer imprint is published by the registered company Springer Nature Switzerland AG
The registered company address is: Gewerbestrasse 11, 6330 Cham, Switzerland

Preface

Ocular inflammation is not at all romantic. In fact, few ophthalmologists like it at all. Even fewer choose to devote careers studying the subject and caring for patients with it. Those who have invested their intellect, time, and energy in the conception of this work are the unusual few who derive great pleasure from diagnosing and treating ocular inflammatory diseases. It is our hope that this book can help other eye care professionals in taking on the challenge of managing patients with uveitis.

Waltham, MA, USA C. Stephen Foster, MD, FACS, FACR

Contents

Contributors

Khawla Abusamra, MD Department of Neurology, University of Kentucky Medical Center, Lexington, KY, USA (Chapters 36, 41, 70)

Aniruddha Agarwal, MD Department of Ophthalmology, Post Graduate Institute of Medical Education and Research (PGIMER), Chandigarh, India (Chapters 12, 27, 44, 50)

Miriam Baron Barshak, MD Department of Medicine, Massachusetts General Hospital, Massachusetts Eye and Ear Infirmary, Harvard Medical School, Boston, MA, USA (Chapters 27, 30, 31, 42, 43, 46, 51)

Pooja V. Bhat, MD Illinois Eye and Ear Infirmary, Department of Ophthalmology and Visual Sciences, University of Illinois at Chicago, Chicago, IL, USA (Chapters 40, 47)

Peter Y. Chang, MD Massachusetts Eye Research and Surgery Institution, Ocular Immunology and Uveitis Foundation, Waltham, MA, USA (Chapters 1)

David S. Chu, MD Rutgers University, Institute of Ophthalmology and Visual Science, Newark, NJ, USA (Chapters 16, 32)

Metropolitan Eye Research and Surgery Institute, Palisades Park, NJ, USA

Christopher D. Conrady, MD, PhD University of Michigan, Kellogg Eye Center – Ophthalmology and Visual Sciences, Ann Arbor, MI, USA (Chapters 21, 48)

Mark Dacey, MD Uveitis Service, Colorado Retina Associates, P.C, Denver, CO, USA (Chapter 23)

Laura Eggenschwiler, MD Department of Ophthalmology, University Hospital Basel, Basel, Switzerland (Chapter 6)

May Ibrahim El Rashedy, MD, PhD Department of Ophthalmology, Cairo University Hospitals, Cairo, Egypt (Chapters 10, 15)

Artur Filipowicz, DO Massachusetts Eye Research and Surgery Institution, Waltham, MA, USA (Chapters 17, 28, 45, 46, 52, 54)

Muhammad Hassan, MD Department of Ophthalmology, Byers Eye Institute, Stanford University, Palo Alto, CA, USA (Chapters 12, 57)

Boonsiri Hunchangsith, MD Banphaeo Eye Hospital (Public Organization), Banphaeo, Thailand (Chapters 11, 26, 60)

Samendra Karkhur, MD Department of Ophthalmology, All India Institute of Medical Sciences, Bhopal, Bhopal, India (Chapters 57)

Mahmut Kaya, MD Department of Ophthalmology, Dokuz Eylul University, Izmir, Turkey (Chapters 7, 33, 39, 49)

Miaoli Lin, MD, PhD C-MER (Shenzhen) Dennis Lam Eye Hospital, Shenzhen, Guangdong, China (Chapter 22)

Arash Maleki, MD Massachusetts Eye Research and Surgery Institution, Waltham, MA, USA (Chapters 4, 29)

Kayla N. Moses, BA Massachusetts Eye Research and Surgery Institution, Waltham, MA, USA (Chapters 5, 18, 51, 59, 61)

Quan Dong Nguyen, MD, MSc Department of Ophthalmology, Byers Eye Institute, Stanford University, Palo Alto, CA, USA (Chapters 12, 57)

Marina Peskina, MD Massachusetts Eye Research and Surgery Institution, Waltham, MA, USA (Chapters 9, 25)

Ravand Samaeekia Illinois Eye and Ear Infirmary, Department of Ophthalmology and Visual Sciences, University of Illinois at Chicago, Chicago, IL, USA (Chapters 40, 47)

Zeynep Seymen, MD, FEBO Department of Ophthalmology, Istanbul Training and Research Hospital, Istanbul, Turkey (Chapters 22, 55)

Yael Sharon Metropolitan Eye Research and Surgery Institute, Palisades Park, NJ, USA (Chapters 16, 32)

Department of Ophthalmology, Rabin Medical Center, Petah-Tikva, Israel

Karen Wingartz Small, MD Professional Eye Care, Mission of Sight, Jamaica, Chattanooga, TN, USA (Chapters 14, 19, 20, 23, 24, 30, 33, 37, 38, 42, 43, 53, 56, 58, 62, 70)

Andrew Phillips Stephenson, BS University of Cincinnati College of Medicine, Cincinnati, OH, USA (Chapters 34, 35)

Anh N. T. Tran, BS Department of Ophthalmology, Spencer Center for Vision Research, Byers Eye Institute, Stanford University, Palo Alto, CA, USA (Chapter 57)

Koushik Tripathy, MD, FRCS (Glasgow) Department of Vitreoretina and Uvea, ASG Eye Hospital, Kolkata, West Bengal, India (Chapters 27, 44, 50)

Jordan A. Ueberroth, MD Massachusetts Eye Research and Surgery Institution, Waltham, MA, USA (Chapters 8, 13, 31, 61, 63, 64, 65, 66, 67, 68, 69, 71)

Albert T. Vitale, MD Department of Ophthalmology and Visual Sciences, University of Utah, Salt Lake City, UT, USA (Chapters 21, 48)

Howard S. Ying, MD, PhD Boston Eye Care Center, Cambridge, MA, USA (Chapters 2, 3)

Catherine Q. Zhu, BS Boston University School of Medicine, Boston, MA, USA (Chapters 2, 3)

1 Diagnosis Flowchart

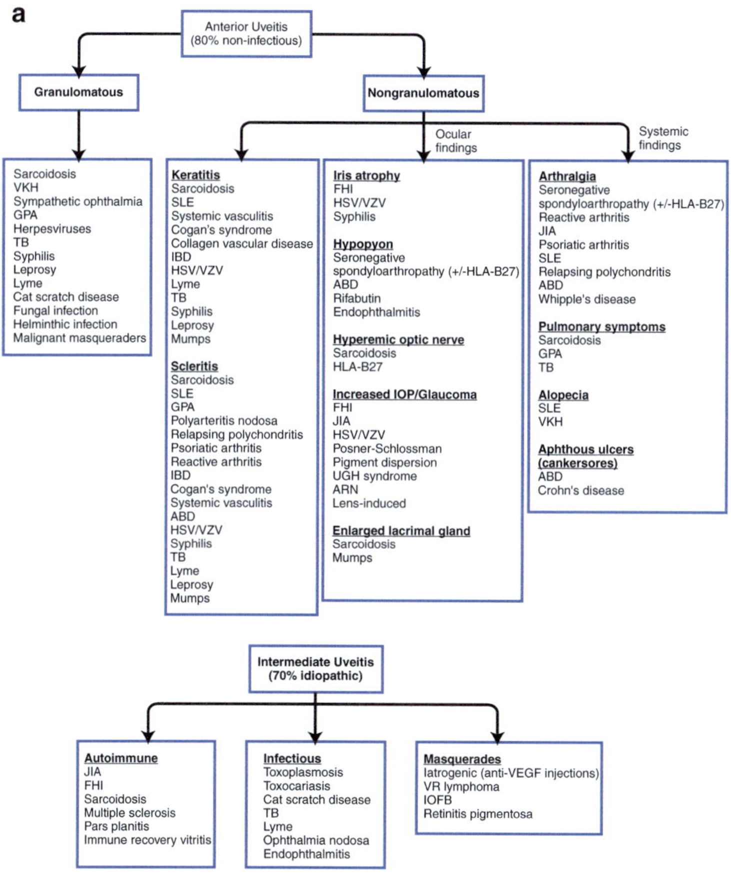

C. S. Foster et al. (eds.), *Uveitis*, https://doi.org/10.1007/978-3-030-52974-1_1

b

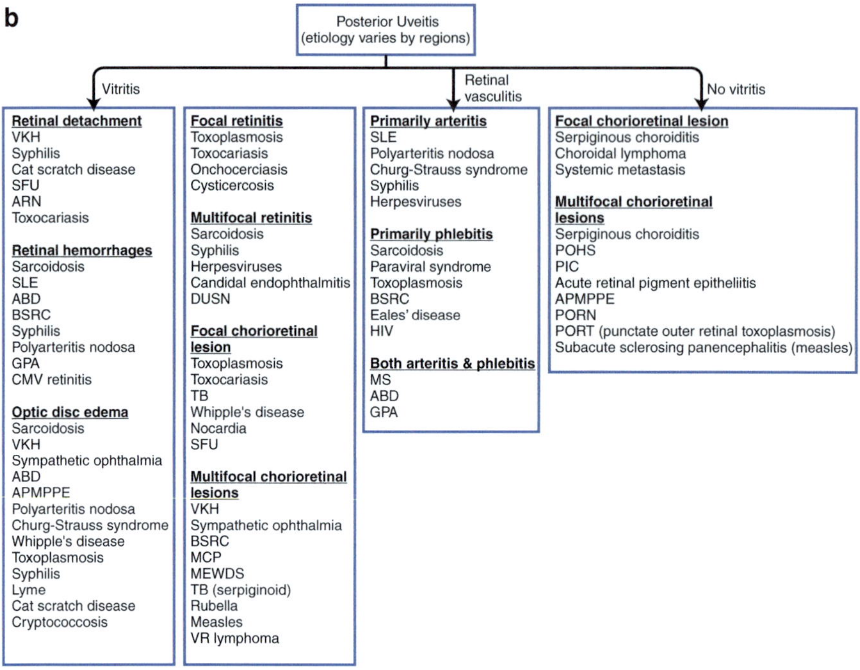
Posterior Uveitis
(etiology varies by regions)
Vitritis
Retinal vasculitis
No vitritis
Retinal detachment
VKH
Syphilis
Cat scratch disease
SFU
ARN
Toxocariasis
Retinal hemorrhages
Sarcoidosis
SLE
ABD
BSRC
Syphilis
Polyarteritis nodosa
GPA
CMV retinitis
Optic disc edema
Sarcoidosis
VKH
Sympathetic ophthalmia
ABD
APMPPE
Polyarteritis nodosa
Churg-Strauss syndrome
Whipple's disease
Toxoplasmosis
Syphilis
Lyme
Cat scratch disease
Cryptococcosis
Focal retinitis
Toxoplasmosis
Toxocariasis
Onchocerciasis
Cysticercosis
Multifocal retinitis
Sarcoidosis
Syphilis
Herpesviruses
Candidal endophthalmitis
DUSN
Focal chorioretinal lesion
Toxoplasmosis
Toxocariasis
TB
Whipple's disease
Nocardia
SFU
Multifocal chorioretinal lesions
VKH
Sympathetic ophthalmia
BSRC
MCP
MEWDS
TB (serpiginoid)
Rubella
Measles
VR lymphoma
Primarily arteritis
SLE
Polyarteritis nodosa
Churg-Strauss syndrome
Syphilis
Herpesviruses
Primarily phlebitis
Sarcoidosis
Paraviral syndrome
Toxoplasmosis
BSRC
Eales' disease
HIV
Both arteritis & phlebitis
MS
ABD
GPA
Focal chorioretinal lesion
Serpiginous choroiditis
Choroidal lymphoma
Systemic metastasis
Multifocal chorioretinal lesions
Serpiginous choroiditis
POHS
PIC
Acute retinal pigment epitheliitis
APMPPE
PORN
PORT (punctate outer retinal toxoplasmosis)
Subacute sclerosing panencephalitis (measles)

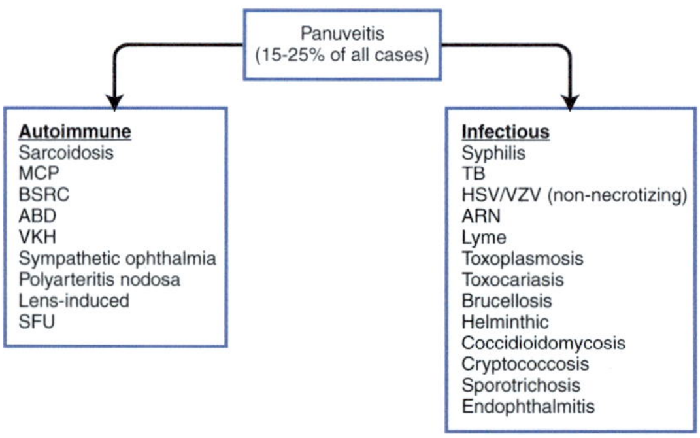
Panuveitis
(15-25% of all cases)
Autoimmune
Sarcoidosis
MCP
BSRC
ABD
VKH
Sympathetic ophthalmia
Polyarteritis nodosa
Lens-induced
SFU
Infectious
Syphilis
TB
HSV/VZV (non-necrotizing)
ARN
Lyme
Toxoplasmosis
Toxocariasis
Brucellosis
Helminthic
Coccidioidomycosis
Cryptococcosis
Sporotrichosis
Endophthalmitis

Seronegative Spondyloarthropathies

2

Overview

- Definition
  - A group of disorders characterized by inflammation of the spine, pelvis, or peripheral joints, lack of RF positivity, and association of the HLA-B27 haplotype
  - Tendency for ocular inflammation (typically anterior uveitis, AU)
  - Includes
    - Ankylosing spondylitis (AS)
    - Reactive arthritis (ReA) (formerly Reiter's syndrome)
    - Psoriatic arthritis (PsA)
    - Enteropathic arthritis (EA) including inflammatory bowel disease (IBD)
      - Whipple's disease, a similar separate infectious entity with some reported association with HLA-B27
    - Juvenile-onset spondyloarthropathies (JSA)
- Symptoms
  - Ocular pain
  - Redness
  - Blurred vision
  - Photophobia
  - Headaches
- Laterality
  - Typically unilateral, alternating
  - Occasionally bilateral (more commonly with IBD)
- Course
  - Acute and recurrent, though IBD associated uveitis may be insidious
  - Uveitis may significantly worsen 1–2 weeks after initial symptoms (delayed severity)

C. S. Foster et al. (eds.), *Uveitis*, https://doi.org/10.1007/978-3-030-52974-1_2

- Age of onset
  - AS: 20–30 years
  - ReA: 18–40 years
  - PsA: 30–40 years, but may occur in young children and elderly
  - EA/IBD: 25–45 years
  - JSA: 9–11 years, psoriasis often before arthritis
- Gender/race
  - AS: M > F; mainly Caucasians; rare in Japanese and black Africans
  - ReA: M > F
  - PsA: M > F
  - EA/IBD: M = F
  - JSA: F > M; girls with more chronic AU, and boys more severe
- Systemic association
  - AS: chronic, systemic disease; inflammation of both sacroiliac joints and the spine
  - ReA: triad of migratory arthritis, urethritis, and conjunctivitis
  - PsA: triad of psoriasis (skin and/or nail); chronic, recurrent erosive polyarthritis (peripheral and/or spinal), and negative RF
  - EA/IBD: arthritis induced by or occurs with IBD (Crohn's disease, ulcerative colitis (UC))
  - JSA: subset of juvenile idiopathic arthritis (JIA) affecting children under age 16, often spanning through adult life

Exam: Ocular

Anterior Segment

- Anterior chamber reaction:
  - Acute onset (may be insidious in IBD)
  - Non-granulomatous, usually mild to moderate cell and flare
  - May progress to hypopyon with plasmoid aqueous, rarely hemorrhage
- Posterior synechiae and cataract are common
- Less common findings:
  - Scleritis: variable diffuse anterior scleritis
  - Conjunctivitis: mild, may be bilateral, non- or micro-purulent, self-limiting
  - Episcleritis: simple or nodular, common in IBD, especially Crohn's
  - Keratitis: typically with conjunctivitis or anterior chamber reaction, fine- to medium-size whitish-gray non-granulomatous endothelial keratic precipitates

Posterior Segment

- Involvement is less common, but may include:
  - Vitritis
  - Multifocal granulomatous choroidal infiltrates
  - Cystoid macular edema
  - Retinal vasculitis
  - Serous retinal detachment
  - Papillitis
  - Retrobulbar neuritis
- Secondary glaucoma is common

Exam: Systemic

- AS:
  - Progressive dull low back pain and stiffness
  - Peripheral arthritis
  - Ankylosing of sacroiliac joints and spine
  - Extra-articular systemic manifestations rare, may present after years
- ReA:
  - Articular involvement within 1 month of inciting urethritis or diarrhea
  - Chronic or recurrent
  - Typically acute onset, migratory, asymmetric, and oligoarticular
  - Arthritis: lower extremity joints most commonly affected
    Sacroiliitis (20–30%) and spondylitis more common in severe disease
    Also dactylitis ("sausage digits"), Achilles tendonitis, plantar fasciitis, calcaneal periostitis, or chest wall pain
  - Genitourinary: urethritis
    Men: prostatitis, seminal vesiculitis, epididymitis, cystitis, or orchitis
    Women: cervicitis and vaginitis
  - Mucocutaneous lesions (>50%) including circinate balanitis, keratoderma blennorrhagicum, oral mucosal lesions, and nail changes
- PsA:
  - Articular involvement may affect any joint
  - Skin lesions with no distinct pattern
  - Nail changes: onycholysis, pitting, ridging, nail discoloration, fragmentation
  - Diffuse swelling of digits, dactylitis ("sausage digits")
- EA/IBD:
  - Peripheral arthritis typically months to years after IBD onset, rarely before
    Usually acute, affecting knees and ankles

- JSA:
  - Less prominent inflammatory back pain
  - Hip and peripheral arthritis
  - Enthesitis

Imaging

- OCT
  - CME
- FA/ICG
  - CME
  - Retinal vasculitis
  - Papillitis
  - Choroidal involvement

Laboratory and Radiographic Testing

- HLA-B27 association, strongly suggestive but not necessarily diagnostic
- Radiographic confirmation of joint damage (plain film radiography, MRI)
- IBD diagnosed by tissue biopsy from colonoscopy
  - Crohn's: granuloma formation with transmural inflammation
  - UC: microabscesses of crypts of Lieberkühn and macroscopic ulcerations with inflammation limited to mucosa

Differential Diagnosis

- Idiopathic
- JIA
- Sarcoidosis
- Adamantiades–Behçet's disease
- Systemic lupus erythematosus
- Tubular interstitial nephritis and uveitis (TINU)
- Infectious:
  - Tuberculosis
  - Viral disease: HSV, EBV
  - Syphilis
  - Whipple's disease
- Pigment dispersion syndrome

Treatment

- Acute AU: frequent topical corticosteroid +/− cycloplegic
  - Initial frequent topical therapy to guard against delayed severity
- Severe AU /posterior involvement: (one or more of the following)
  - Frequent topical corticosteroid (q1-2h)
  - Atropine 1% BID with severe plasmoid AC reaction, hypopyon
  - Periorbital corticosteroid injection 40 mg/mL (sub-Tenon's, trans-septal)
  - Oral corticosteroid with taper
- Posterior involvement similar to severe AU with element to treat posterior disease
- Severe, recurrent, chronic: step-ladder steroid-sparing immunomodulatory therapy
  - NSAIDs for mild disease without CME
  - Chemo/biologics for more significant disease
  - Systemic involvement may drive therapy

Referral/Co-management

- Rheumatology
- Gastroenterology
- Pediatrics

3 Systemic Lupus Erythematosus

Overview

- Definition
  - Chronic, multisystem, autoimmune disease characterized by the production of numerous autoantibodies, mostly targeted against components of the cell nuclei
  - Damage is mediated by immune complex deposition in tissues (lupus nephritis and arthritis) or by direct effects of auto-Ab on cell surface molecules or serum components (hemolytic anemia, thrombocytopenia, antiphospholipid syndrome)
  - Disease severity and prognosis vary widely depending on the extent of organ involvement
- Symptoms
  - May precede systemic presentation
  - Wide ranging from dry eye symptoms, ocular pain and photosensitivity, to severe loss of vision
- Laterality
  - Can present unilaterally or bilaterally
- Course
  - Relapsing and remitting
- Age of onset
  - Typically late teens to early 40s, but 15% have late onset (late 50s–early 60s)
- Gender/race
  - F:M = 9:1
  - African Americans, Asians, and Hispanics are more affected
- Systemic association
  - Skin, joints, and kidneys are classically involved, but practically all organs can be affected, as the autoantibodies target all cellular nuclei
  - Skin (85% of patients): butterfly rash across the nose and cheeks, known as malar flush, is the most common finding. Other findings include discoid rash (erythematous raised areas with adherent keratotic scaling and follicular

C. S. Foster et al. (eds.), *Uveitis*, https://doi.org/10.1007/978-3-030-52974-1_3

Table 3.1 The American College of Rheumatology Criteria for SLE

Malar rash
Discoid rash
Photosensitivity
Oral ulcers
Arthritis (nonerosive, 2 or more peripheral joints)
Serositis (pleuritis, pericarditis)
Renal disorders (proteinuria, nephritis)
Neurologic disorder (seizures, psychosis)
Hematologic disorder (hemolytic anemia, leukopenia, lymphopenia, thrombocytopenia)
Immunologic disorder (positive LE cell prep, anti-native DNA, anti-Sm, false-positive test for syphilis)
Antinuclear antibody in the absence of drugs associated with drug-induced lupus

plugging), cutaneous ulcers, splinter hemorrhages, purpuric skin lesions, and alopecia

- Musculoskeletal (85%): painful peripheral joints, non-deforming migratory polyarthritis, myalgia, and myositis
- Renal (50%): the major cause of morbidity and mortality in SLE patients; manifest as nephrotic syndrome, mesangial disease, focal or diffuse proliferative nephritis, and membranous glomerulonephritis
- Painless oral ulcers (30–40%)
- Neuropsychiatric (30%): seizures, organic brain syndrome, psychosis; transverse myelitis is rare (4%) but is associated with optic neuritis
- Raynaud's phenomenon (20%)
- Cardiac (20%): pericarditis, myocarditis, Libman-Sacks endocarditis (also known as nonbacterial thrombotic endocarditis + phospholipid antibody)
- Pulmonary: pleuritis and pneumonitis
- Hepatosplenomegaly and adenopathy are common despite not being part of diagnostic criteria (see Table 3.1)
- Hematologic: chronic anemia, hemolytic anemia, leukopenia, lymphopenia, thrombocytopenia, and increased thrombotic risks
- Secondary antiphospholipid syndrome (APL): deep vein thrombosis, cerebral arterial thrombosis, pulmonary embolism, thrombocytopenia, and recurrent fetal loss (typically in second and third trimesters) in the presence of APL antibodies

Exam: Ocular

External

- Discoid rash: erythematosus rash over the eyelids characterized by keratotic scaling and follicular plugging (may coexist with blepharitis and thus be overlooked)
- Strabismus due to cranial nerve or muscle involvement

Anterior Segment

- Keratoconjunctivitis sicca
- Episcleritis: generally benign and self-limiting
- Scleritis: anterior diffuse or nodular scleritis; necrotizing is rare
- Recurrent corneal erosions, peripheral keratitis (ulcerative or not), interstitial keratitis, endotheliitis
- Anterior uveitis is rare, non-granulomatous, and typically mild

Posterior Segment

- Retinopathy is the most well-recognized ocular manifestation of SLE, observed in 1 out of 10 patients
  - Microangiopathy is an extremely accurate barometer of systemic disease activity: cotton-wool spots (most common), arteriolar attenuation, retinal hemorrhage, microaneurysms
  - Retinal findings are compounded by systemic hypertension as a sequelae of SLE nephropathy: AV nicking, hard exudates, papilledema, and multifocal choroidal infarctions (Elschnig's spots)
  - Occlusive vasculitis affects the arterioles primarily, causing vascular sheathing and retinal opacification; diffuse non-perfusion leads to neovascular complications such as vitreous hemorrhage, tractional retinal detachment, and glaucoma
  - Venous occlusion is less common and may be due to venous stasis secondary to arterial occlusion
- Choroidopathy is uncommon
  - Present as single or multifocal serous retinal detachment
  - Associated with CNS vasculitis, nephropathy, and uncontrolled hypertension
  - Very responsive to systemic therapy
- Vitritis is rare
- Optic nerve involvement
  - Papillitis due to optic nerve vasculitis
  - Optic neuritis with resultant ischemic optic neuropathy; transverse myelitis is seen in more than half of these patients
  - Papilledema from rare pseudotumor cerebri

Exam: Systemic

- For clinical research, at least 4 of 11 ACR diagnostic criteria need to be met (Table 3.1). However, in practice, patients with fewer than 4 can still be diagnosed with SLE

Imaging

- OCT
  - Macular edema
  - Subretinal fluid in choroidopathy
- FA
  - Microaneurysms
  - Retinal non-perfusion with retinal neovascularization
  - Macular leakage
  - Optic nerve leakage
- ICG
  - Early, transient hypofluorescence followed by late hyperfluorescence in areas of choroidopathy
  - Multifocal hyperfluorescence during intermediate phase possibly indicative of immune complex staining

Laboratory and Radiographic Testing

- BMP, CBC, LFTs, and complete urinalysis
- ANA: nonspecific but present in almost all patients (97–98%); diffuse, peripheral or speckled pattern
- Anti-dsDNA and anti-Smith antibodies are most SLE-specific
  - Anti-dsDNA Ab: present in 30% of SLE patients, tends to represent a more serious disease state such as nephritis; however, its level cannot be used to monitor disease activity
  - Anti-Sm Ab: present in 20% of SLE patients; does not reflect disease severity
- Less SLE-specific antibodies: anti-Ro/SSA and anti-La/SSB (30–40%), anti-U1RNP (25%), APL (17%)
- Anti-histone Abs typically suggests drug-induced SLE, but may also be found in primary SLE
- Total complement (CH50), C3, C4 can be low due to complement consumption
- Chest X-ray
- Echocardiogram

Differential Diagnosis

- Adamantiades-Behcet's disease
- Polyarteritis nodosa
- Takayasu's disease
- Granulomatosis with polyangiitis (Wegener's)
- Syphilis

Treatment

- Oral NSAIDs and aminoquinolines, including chloroquine and hydroxychloroquine, may be appropriate for cutaneous lupus, arthritis, and serositis
- Systemic corticosteroids are reserved for hematologic, renal, and CNS diseases; long-term steroid-sparing immunosuppression may be necessary in systemic and ocular lupus (ocular flare-up can occur despite systemic quiescence)
- Plasmapheresis in combination with immunosuppressive therapy has been used in a few severe, recalcitrant cases
- Laser photocoagulation +/− intravitreal anti-VEGF are used in severe vaso-occlusive disease to prevent ischemic complications

Referral/Co-management

- Rheumatology
- Nephrology
- Other specialists per systemic involvement

4 Scleroderma

- Definition
  - An autoimmune, multisystem connective tissue disease characterized by severe inflammation and excessive deposition of collagen and other intracellular materials in the skin and internal organs
  - Localized scleroderma: most common; patchy skin involvement
  - Systemic scleroderma: limited or diffuse

    Limited form: formerly *CREST* syndrome
    - *C*alcinosis (calcium deposition in the skin)
    - *R*aynaud's phenomenon
    - *E*sophageal dysmotility
    - *S*clerodactyly (skin tightening of the fingers)
    - *T*elangiectasia (of the skin)

    Diffuse form: most serious and life-threatening
    - Lungs, heart, and kidneys also involved with skin
  - Ocular involvement rare

    Dry eyes, ocular surface changes, uveitis, glaucoma
- Symptoms
  - Decreased vision
  - Redness
  - Itching, burning
  - Foreign body sensation
  - Tearing
  - Ocular pain
  - Photophobia
  - Floaters
- Laterality
  - Bilateral, but can be asymmetric

C. S. Foster et al. (eds.), *Uveitis*, https://doi.org/10.1007/978-3-030-52974-1_4

- Course
  - Chronic with high mortality rate in cases with extensive skin, pulmonary and renal involvement
  - Not typically progressive; disease may plateau
- Age of onset
  - 35–55 years with peak incidence in the fifth decade
  - Pediatric form also exists
- Gender/race
  - F:M = 3:1
  - Worldwide prevalence, more common in blacks than whites
- Systemic association
  - Skin is always the first organ involved
  - Variable subsequent involvement of internal organs including lungs, kidneys, heart

Exam: Ocular

- *External*
  - Skin tightness with lid eversion and blepharophimosis
  - Lid telangiectasia in 20% of patients
  - Extraocular myopathy
- *Anterior segment*
  - Common findings:
    - Decreased tear meniscus and keratoconjunctivitis sicca
    - Subepithelial fibrosis, shortening of fornices
    - Conjunctival vascularization, vessel varicosities, telangiectasia, and loss of fine conjunctival vessels
  - Less common findings:
    - Scleral pits
    - Exposure keratopathy, peripheral ulcerative keratitis, pellucid marginal degeneration, keratomalacia
    - Iris transillumination defect
    - Anterior uveitis (granulomatous or non-granulomatous) rare
- *Posterior segment*
  - Less common findings:
    - Vitritis
    - Glaucomatous and non-glaucomatous optic neuropathy
    - Retinal vein occlusion with retinal hemorrhage, cotton wool spots, parafoveal telangiectasia, and macular edema
    - Choroiditis resulting in patchy choroidal non-perfusion with secondary choriocapillaris and RPE atrophy

Exam: Systemic

- *Skin*
  - Increased capillary size on nail fold points to systemic scleroderma
  - Symmetric painless swelling and thickening of fingers, hands, sometimes feet and ankles
  - Raynaud phenomenon
  - Skin atrophy, telangiectasia, and calcinosis are late signs
  - Reduced oral aperture due to perioral fibrosis
- *Internal organs*
  - Kidney, lung, heart, and gastrointestinal systems can also be involved especially in diffuse systemic scleroderma

Imaging

- OCT
  - Macular edema
  - RPE and choroidal atrophy
  - Thickened choroid during active choroiditis, as seen on enhanced depth imaging EDI-OCT
- FA
  - Microvascular changes in retinal vasculature may lead to patches of hyper- and hypo-fluorescent areas
  - Retinal vein occlusion leading to retinal non-perfusion, telangiectasia, and macular leakage
- ICG
  - Hypercyanescence, "hazy" choroidal vessels, indicates choroiditis

Laboratory and Radiographic Testing

- Urinalysis
- ANA (positive in 90%)
- Scleroderma-specific ANAs
  - Anti-topoisomerase-1 and anti-SCL-70 Abs for diffuse systemic scleroderma
  - Anti-centromere Abs for limited systemic scleroderma
- Chest X-ray
- Barium swallow

Differential Diagnosis

- Nephrogenic systemic fibrosis
- Graft-versus-host disease
- Porphyria cutanea tarda

- Sjögren's syndrome
- Dermatomyositis
- Diabetic cheiroarthropathy (limited joint mobility)
- Eosinophilic fasciitis

Treatment

Systemic

- Raynaud's phenomenon
  - Dihydropyridine-type calcium channel blockers (e.g., nifedipine) and prostanoids (e.g., iloprost)
- Gastrointestinal symptoms
  - Proton-pump inhibitors for acid reflux prevention
  - Prokinetics for dysmotility
  - Rotating antibiotics for bacterial overgrowth
- Renal crisis
  - ACE inhibitors
- Pulmonary hypertension
  - Endothelin receptor antagonists (bosentan)
  - Selective endothelin-A receptor antagonists (ambrisentan)
  - Phosphodiesterase inhibitors (sildenafil)
  - Intravenous prostacyclins (epoprostenol)
  - Cyclophosphamide for interstitial lung disease

Ocular

- Dry eyes
  - Artificial tears, topical cyclosporine A, serum tears, and punctal occlusion
- Lid lesions
  - Topical corticosteroid cream
- Ocular myopathy
  - Oral corticosteroids
- Uveitis
  - Appropriate topical, regional, or oral corticosteroid therapy for acute flares
  - Steroid sparing immunomodulatory therapy for chronic disease
    - Oral, SC, or IV antimetabolites, biologics
    - B cell depletion such as rituximab and BAFF (B-cell activating factor) blocking agents
    - Cyclosporine avoided due to renal toxicity

Referral/Co-management

- Dermatology
- Nephrology
- Cardiology
- Pulmonology

Fuchs' Heterochromic Iridocyclitis

5

Overview

- Definition
  - Low-grade, chronic but intermittent, often self-limiting non-granulomatous anterior uveitis
  - Commonly felt to be of occult infectious origin, specifically rubella virus (Toxoplasma and CMV have also been suspected, but not shown)
- Symptoms
  - Blurring
  - Floaters
  - Redness and pain are less common
  - May be asymptomatic
- Laterality
  - Mostly unilateral (10% bilateral)
- Course
  - Mild
  - Chronic, fluctuating over time
- Age of onset
  - All ages, though most present in early adulthood
- Gender/race
  - No predilection
- Systemic association
  - None

C. S. Foster et al. (eds.), *Uveitis*, https://doi.org/10.1007/978-3-030-52974-1_5

Exam: Ocular

Anterior Segment

- Mild iridocyclitis
- Diffuse iris stromal atrophy (with or without heterochromia)
- Also common
  - Keratic precipitates, may be stellate
  - General lack of posterior synechiae, prior to cataract surgery
  - Cataract
  - Elevated IOP
  - Iris nodules

    Busacca – stromal

    Koeppe – pupillary margin.
  - Endothelial changes
- Less common
  - Corneal edema (with elevated IOP)
  - Russell bodies – minute, crystalline, highly refractile iris deposits
  - Angle neovascularization
  - Hyphema after anterior chamber paracentesis (due to angle vessels)

Posterior Segment

- Cells or opacities in anterior vitreous
- Glaucomatous optic neuropathy (up to 59%)
- Cystoid macular edema is NOT seen
- Scattered peripheral focal chorioretinal scars
  - Variable, may be bilateral

Exam: Systemic

- No associated findings

Imaging

- Corneal confocal microscopy: endothelial infiltrate, spotlike holes, enlarged intercellular boundaries
- FA: anterior segment angiography may highlight increased angle or iris vessels

Laboratory and Radiographic Testing

- No definitive serologic or laboratory testing
- Aqueous studies
  - Rubella IgG
  - PCR for viral DNA (HSV, VZV, CMV)

Differential Diagnosis

- Herpetic iridocyclitis
  - Typically sectoral iris atrophy, not diffuse
- Posner-Schlossman syndrome (glaucomatocyclitis crisis)
- Neovascular glaucoma
- Toxoplasmosis
- Sarcoidosis

Treatment

- Low-potency topical corticosteroids used as needed or as maintenance therapy
  - May help to lower IOP during active inflammation
- Systemic medications are of no benefit
- Medical or surgical glaucoma care as needed
- Perioperative topical corticosteroids

Referral/Co-management

- None

Sarcoidosis

6

Overview

- Definition
  - Multisystem non-caseating granulomatous disease of unknown etiology
  - Ocular involvement in 30%, mostly chronic granulomatous anterior uveitis, but may involve posterior structures, retinal vessels, optic nerve
  - Criteria for ocular sarcoidosis:
    - Definite – uveitis with biopsy positive
    - Presumed – uveitis with bilateral hilar lymphadenopathy (BHL), no biopsy
    - Probable – 3 suggestive intraocular signs *and* 2 labs, BHL negative, no biopsy done
    - Possible – 4 suggestive intraocular signs *and* 2 labs, biopsy negative
- Symptoms
  - Blurring
  - Redness
  - Floaters, flashes
  - Pain, irritation
    - May be deep orbital pain
  - Photophobia
  - Scotomas
  - Diplopia (with orbital involvement)
- Laterality
  - Unilateral or bilateral
- Course
  - Acute or chronic

C. S. Foster et al. (eds.), *Uveitis*, https://doi.org/10.1007/978-3-030-52974-1_6

- Age of onset
  - Two peaks of incidence:
    - 20s to 30s (typically acute form)
    - 50s to 60s (typically chronic form)
  - Early onset sarcoidosis (first decade) is actually sporadic form of Blau syndrome (*NOD2* mutation)
- Gender/race
  - No specific gender predilection, but females may have more eye and neurologic involvement
  - More common in US blacks (often presents earlier, more severe) and northern European whites
  - Less common in Asians
- Systemic association
  - Multisystem non-caseating granulomas involving one or several organ systems including primarily lungs, but also lymph nodes (hilar and mediastinal most common), eyes, skin, heart, joints, spleen, liver, and nervous system
  - Hypercalcemia
  - Ocular symptoms may precede systemic signs

Exam: Ocular

Anterior Segment

- Granulomatous anterior uveitis (22–70%)
  - Bilateral, chronic
  - Mutton-fat keratic precipitates
    - May also present with fine keratic precipitates
- More common
  - Conjunctival nodules (variable %)
    - Solitary, yellow, "millet-seed," often on bulbar surface
  - Posterior synechiae
  - Iris nodules
    - Busacca (iris stroma)
    - Koeppe (pupil margin)
  - Peripheral anterior synechiae
  - Cataract
  - Orbital inflammation, myositis, lacrimal gland enlargement
  - Nasolacrimal duct obstruction
- Less common
  - Band keratopathy
    - Associated with hypercalcemia
  - Scleritis (rare), anterior or posterior
    - Angle closure (due to annular ciliochoroidal detachment)

Posterior Segment

- Vitritis or intermediate uveitis
  - Inferior vitreous (snowballs*) or pars plana exudates (snowbank*)
  - * not to be confused with inactive fibrotic changes along pars plana
  - String of pearls – vitreous exudate strands in chains
  - May also be posterior uveitis or panuveitis
- Cystoid macular edema
- Retinal vasculitis (very common)
  - Segmental phlebitis
  - "Taches de bougie" or candle wax drippings
    - Creamy white perivascular exudate or sheathing
- Papillitis (may be only posterior manifestation)
- Retinal vein occlusion
  - Ischemic retinopathy with neovascularization, less common
- Glaucoma
- Choroidal nodules
- Multifocal punctate mid-peripheral chorioretinal scars
  - "Punched-out lesions," very characteristic
- Choroidal neovascularization, peripapillary or subfoveal
- Exudative retinal detachment (less common)
  - Posterior scleritis with annular ciliochoroidal detachment (angle closure)

Exam: Systemic

- Acute disease (weeks)
  - Fever, erythema nodosum, arthralgia, parotid enlargement
- Pulmonary (90%)
  - Hilar and mediastinal lymphadenopathy
    - Mediastinal without hilar LAD is rare, alternative diagnosis
  - Pulmonary nodules
  - Calcification
  - May also involve upper respiratory mucosa
- Skin (9–37%)
  - Erythema nodosum
  - Plaque-like lesions
    - Lupus pernio – indurated, chronic violaceous, often on face
  - Subcutaneous nodules
  - Glandular enlargement (salivary, parotitis)
- Neurologic (5–26%)
  - May involve any part of nervous system
    - Occurs in 37% of patients with ocular involvement
  - Cranial neuropathies, most common
  - Hypothalamic or pituitary lesions may lead to endocrinologic disease

  - Meningeal
  - Spinal cord
- Cardiac (up to 25%)
  - Cardiomyopathy
  - Pericardial effusion or pericarditis
  - Conduction abnormalities
  - Cor pulmonale (with severe pulmonary disease)
- Hepatosplenic enlargement with granulomas/nodules (>50%)
- Musculoskeletal
  - Arthritis – ankles, other joints
  - Bone resorption in marrow of phalanges
- Renal (uncommon)
  - Interstitial nephritis
  - Calculus
  - Renal failure

Imaging

- OCT: CME, disc edema
- ED-OCT: choroidal granuloma
- OCT-A: retinal ischemia, microvascular disease
- FA: venule (very common) or capillary leakage or staining, CME, diffuse chorioretinal leakage, disc leakage, peripapillary or subfoveal choroidal neovascularization, ischemia, retinal vein occlusion, choroidal granuloma
- ICG: early lobular hypolucence, choroidal vasculitis, focal and diffuse late hyperlucence
- VF: glaucoma, optic neuropathy, craniopathy
- B-Scan: orbital inflammation, posterior scleritis, choroidal granuloma, papillitis

Laboratory and Radiographic Testing

- ACE or lysozyme may be elevated in active disease, often normal, nonspecific
- Elevated soluble interleukin-2 receptor (sIL2R)
- Hypercalcemia, hypercalciuria
- Chest CT – occult or symptomatic pulmonary findings, cardiomyopathy
  - Chest X-ray often negative, nonspecific
- MRI brain/orbits – CNS involvement, orbital inflammation
- Gallium scan
  - Panda sign – bilateral symmetric lacrimal and parotid uptake
  - Lambda sign – para- and infrahilar bronchopulmonary lymph nodes and right paratracheal (azygous) mediastinal lymph nodes
- Biopsy – conjunctiva, vitreous (high levels of HMGB1), transbronchial lung, lacrimal gland, skin

- Other testing
  - Cutaneous anergy
  - Pulmonary function testing
  - Bronchoalveolar lavage
  - PET imaging

Differential Diagnosis

- Anterior uveitis
  - HLA-B27 associated uveitis
  - Fuchs' heterochromic iridocyclitis
  - Herpes simplex or varicella zoster
  - Syphilis
  - Tuberculosis
  - Juvenile idiopathic arthritis
- Intermediate uveitis
  - Pars planitis
  - Multiple sclerosis
  - Lyme disease
- Posterior uveitis
  - Toxoplasmosis
  - Toxocariasis
  - Tuberculosis
  - Syphilis
  - Birdshot retinochoroidopathy
  - Multifocal choroiditis and panuveitis
  - Vogt-Koyanagi-Harada disease
  - Intraocular lymphoma
  - Sympathetic ophthalmia
  - Adamantiades-Behçet's disease
  - Whipple's disease

Treatment

- Acute AU: frequent topical corticosteroid +/− cycloplegia
  - Q1h steroid and atropine 1% BID with hypopyon
- Severe AU or <u>any</u> posterior involvement
  - Systemic corticosteroids, oral or intravenous
  - Initiation of immunomodulatory therapy
    - Coordination with other specialists if necessary
- Immunomodulatory therapy
  - Antimetabolites
    - Methotrexate particularly effective

    Azathioprine or mycophenolate
  - Calcineurin inhibitors (supplemental)
    Cyclosporine, tacrolimus
  - Biologics (especially with RV)
    TNFα inhibitors – adalimumab, infliximab
    Anti-IL6 - tocilizumab
    CD20 inhibition – rituximab
    Anti-IL1β – anakinra, canakinumab (used in some cases)
  - Alkylating agents
    Chlorambucil or cyclophosphamide
- Intravitreal therapy
  - Anti-VEGF
  - Corticosteroid injections, implants
- Pan-retinal photocoagulation
- Other therapeutic measures
  - Hydroxychloroquine
  - IV-Ig
  - Subcutaneous corticotropin gel
  - Thalidomide

Referral/Co-management

- Pulmonology
- Rheumatology
- Neurology
- Cardiology
- Dermatology
- Endocrinology

7 Adamantiades-Behçet's Disease

Overview

- Definition
  - A chronic, relapsing inflammatory disorder of unknown etiology with classic triad findings
    - Recurrent oral and genital aphthous ulcers
    - Ocular inflammation
    - Skin lesions
  - International criteria:
    - Behçet's Research Committee of Japan
      - Complete, incomplete, suspect, possible
    - International Study Group for Behçet's Disease Criteria
      - Oral ulcers +2 of: genital ulcers, eye lesions, skins lesions, pathergy test
  - Frequently involves CNS and GI tract as well
  - Ocular inflammation in 67–95%
    - Anterior uveitis
    - Devastating retinal vasculitis
- Symptoms
  - Blurring
  - Scotomas
  - Redness
  - Periorbital pain
  - Photophobia
  - Tearing with rare ocular discharge
  - Diplopia (with neurologic involvement)
- Laterality
  - Unilateral progressing to bilateral, 80%

C. S. Foster et al. (eds.), *Uveitis*, https://doi.org/10.1007/978-3-030-52974-1_7

- Course
  - Recurrent inflammation, not typically chronic
  - Ocular flares are often severe
- Age of onset
  - 25–35 years worldwide (range 2 months to 72 years)
- Gender/race
  - Historically M > F, may be more even distribution
  - Most common in Eastern Mediterranean and East Asian
- Systemic association
  - Systemic vasculitis
  - Oral and/or genital aphthous ulcers
  - Various mild to severe organ involvement including skin, heart, CNS, GI, lungs, GU, joints

Exam: Ocular

Anterior Segment

- Acute anterior uveitis (AU):
  - Non-granulomatous
  - May progress to "shifting" hypopyon if untreated, 19–31%
- More common:
  - Cataract
  - Posterior synechiae
  - Peripheral anterior synechiae
  - Iris atrophy
- Less common:
  - Scleritis
  - Episcleritis
  - Filamentary keratitis
  - Neovascularization of iris
    - From posterior inflammation
    - Poor prognostic sign

Posterior Segment

- Posterior or panuveitis
  - Vitritis with acute inflammation
- Retinal and/or vitreous hemorrhage
- Venous and capillary dilatation
- Obliterative necrotizing retinal vasculitis (RV)
  - May involve arteries and veins simultaneously (also capillaries)
  - Ghost vessels, "silver-wired" vessels

  - CRVO or BRVO
  - CRAO or BRAO
  - NVE, NVD
- CME
- Chorioretinal scarring
- Retinal tears and detachment
- Papillitis, later progressive optic atrophy
- Neovascular glaucoma

Exam: Systemic

- Oral aphthous ulcers, required for diagnosis
- Skin
  - Erythema nodosum
  - Hyperpigmented/hypopigmented scarring
  - Pathergy (40%)
  - Acne vulgaris or folliculitis, on thorax or face
- Vasculitis (8–38%)
  - Any vessels (arteries, veins, capillaries), any size
  - Superficial thrombophlebitis, upper or lower extremities
- Neurologic (3–10%, neurologic or vascular in origin)
  - Cranial nerve palsies (CN VI, CN VII, transient)
  - Papillitis, papilledema
  - Audiovestibular dysfunction
  - Venous sinus thromboses, intracranial hypertension
  - Pyramidal brainstem lesions
  - Seizures
  - Psychiatric disorders
- Genitourinary
  - Ulcers
  - Epididymitis
  - Glomerulonephritis
  - IgA nephropathy
  - Amyloidosis
  - Renal vein thrombosis
- Gastrointestinal
  - Diarrhea
  - Hemorrhages
  - Ulcers in esophagus, stomach, intestine; may perforate
- Pulmonary (18%)
  - Hemoptysis, dyspnea, chest pain, fever, cough
  - Vascular lesions, pulmonary emboli
  - Aneurysmal bronchial fistula

- Musculoskeletal
  - Arthritis – knee, sacroiliitis, ankylosing spondylitis, non-migrating

Imaging

- OCT: CME, CNV, macular atrophy (after vascular insult)
- FA: CME, retinal vasculitis (may see arteritis, phlebitis, and/or capillaritis), papillitis, vascular occlusion/delay, neovascularization, chorioretinitis
  - Diffuse dye leakage may be seen after inflammation subsides
- ICG: hypocyanescent choroidal lesions
- ERG: decreases in overall standard and pattern ERG

Laboratory and Radiographic Testing

- No definitive serologic or laboratory testing
- May be elevated acute phase reactant proteins: ESR, CRP, complement
- HLA-B51 association (not diagnostic)
- Elevated soluble CD25 may precede recurrence

Differential Diagnosis

- HLA-B27 associated uveitis
  - Reactive arthritis
- Sarcoidosis
- Systemic lupus erythematosus
- ANCA vasculitides
- Viral retinitis

Treatment

- Acute AU: frequent topical corticosteroid +/− cycloplegia
  - Q1h steroid and atropine 1% BID with hypopyon
- Severe AU or posterior involvement
  - Requires aggressive and urgent therapy
  - Systemic corticosteroids, oral or intravenous (or both)
  - Initiation of immunomodulatory therapy
    - May coordinate with other specialists
- Immunomodulatory therapy
  - Antimetabolites
    - Azathioprine or mycophenolate

  - Calcineurin inhibitors
    Cyclosporine may supplement antimetabolite therapy
  - Biologics (especially with RV)
    TNFα inhibitors – adalimumab, infliximab
    CD20 inhibition – rituximab
    Anti-IL1β – anakinra, canakinumab (used in some cases)
  - Alkylating agents
    Chlorambucil or cyclophosphamide
- Other therapeutic measures
  - Colchicine
  - Plasmapheresis
  - Interferon α-2a
  - Dapsone
  - Pendoxyphilline
  - Penicillin
  - Thalidomide

Referral/Co-management

- Rheumatology
- Cardiology
- Neurology
- Dermatology
- ENT
- Gastroenterology
- Urology
- Pulmonology

Polyarteritis Nodosa

8

Overview

- Definition
  - An uncommon but potentially lethal multisystem nongranulomatous necrotizing vasculitis of small- or medium-sized arteries, principally at branching and bifurcation points.
  - Typically ANCA negative.
  - Associated with certain viral infections (hepatitis B most common), drug abuse, hyposensitization/desensitization treatment, B cell neoplasms, and acute otitis media.
  - Ocular manifestations occur in 10–20% of patients and include necrotizing scleritis, peripheral ulcerative keratitis, uveitis, and choroidal and retinal vasculitis.
- Symptoms
  - Redness
  - Exquisite pain – periorbital or with extraocular movements
  - Photophobia
  - Blurry vision
- Laterality
  - Unilateral or bilateral
- Course
  - Progressive and fatal without treatment due to renal and cardiac complications (5-year mortality rate is 80–95% if untreated)
- Age of onset
  - 40–60 years
- Gender/race
  - M:F = 2:1.
  - No racial predilection *per se*, but polyarteritis nodosa (PAN) has the highest prevalence in Alaskan Eskimo because the population has a very high rate of hepatitis B infection

C. S. Foster et al. (eds.), *Uveitis*, https://doi.org/10.1007/978-3-030-52974-1_8

- Systemic association
- Multisystem involvement tends to occur early
  - Renal (75%)
    Glomerulonephritis, hematuria, hypertension
    Primary cause of death
  - Cardiac (75%)
    Coronary thrombosis, pericarditis, pericardial hemorrhage, acute aortitis.
    Myocardial involvement leads to dysrhythmias and infarction.
    Second leading cause of death.
  - Cutaneous (20–50%)
    Cutaneous or subcutaneous nodules along superficial arteries around the knee, anterior lower leg, and dorsum of foot
    - Nodules can rupture resulting in cutaneous hematomas or ecchymosis.

    Infarction or gangrene involving the fingers or toes
  - Gastrointestinal
    Abdominal pain caused by intestinal or mesenteric ischemia
    Infarcts in the liver and spleen
    Other findings: peritonitis, bowel gangrene and perforation, and intra-abdominal hemorrhage
  - Neurologic
    Ischemia to peripheral nerves, causing mononeuritis multiplex
  - Genitourinary
    Epididymitis: virtually pathognomonic in appropriate clinical context
  - Musculoskeletal
    Non-deforming arthritis
    Myalgia

Exam: Ocular

External

- Orbital inflammation, sometimes causing exophthalmos/proptosis

Anterior Segment

- Conjunctival hyperemia, hemorrhage, or infarction
- Episcleritis
- Necrotizing scleritis with peripheral ulcerative keratitis (most common type of scleritis in PAN)
- Acute nongranulomatous anterior uveitis

Posterior Segment

- Choroidal and retinal vasculitis (most common)
- Exudative retinal detachment
- Vascular occlusion
- Hypertensive retinopathy

Neuro-Ophthalmic Findings

- Optic nerve vasculitis causing optic disc edema
- Vasculitis involving the central and peripheral nervous systems leading to third, fifth, sixth, or seventh cranial nerve palsies, hemianopia, nystagmus, amaurosis fugax, and/or Horner's syndrome

Exam: Systemic

- Cutaneous or subcutaneous nodules along superficial arteries of lower extremities
- Peripheral nerve paresis or paresthesia
- Abdominal tenderness
- Testicular/epididymal tenderness

Imaging

- FA
  - Delayed choroidal filling
  - Retinal arteritis
- ICG
  - Choroidal infarction

Laboratory and Radiographic Testing

- Diagnosis is made on clinical and histological grounds.
  - Biopsy of involved tissue may show hemorrhagic vasculitis and fibrinoid necrosis
  - Testicular and skin biopsy confirm diagnosis in 50–80% of patients
- Hepatitis B panel: 33% have positive surface antigen (HBsAg).
- Other labs are nonspecific and simply reflect the systemic nature of PAN.
  - Elevated ESR/CRP and neutrophil count
  - Hypocomplementemia
  - Elevated BUN and serum creatinine

  - Urinalysis: RBC, red cell casts, or protein
  - p-ANCA is NOT typically associated with PAN, but a subset of PAN called microscopic polyangiitis (involving even smaller vessels) IS associated with p-ANCA
- Abdominal and renal angiography.
  - Saccular arterial aneurysms in renal, hepatic, and gastrointestinal vasculature

Differential Diagnosis

- Systemic vasculitides
  - Granulomatosis with polyangiitis
  - Eosinophilic granulomatosis with polyangiitis (Churg-Strauss)
  - Microscopic polyangiitis
- Rheumatoid arthritis
- Adamantiades-Behcet's disease
- Systemic lupus erythematosus
- Dermatomyositis
- Progressive systemic sclerosis
- Idiopathic retinal vasculitis, aneurysms, and neuroretinitis (IRVAN)
- Syphilis
- Mooren's ulcer (no scleritis)

Treatment

- Prednisone 1 mg/kg/day + cyclophosphamide 1–2 mg/kg/day.
- Biologics in refractory cases, including adalimumab, infliximab, rituximab, tocilizumab, and tofacitinib.
- Treatment of HBV may produce remission.

Referral/Co-management

- Rheumatology
- Nephrology
- Urology
- Cardiology
- Neurology
- Gastroenterology

Granulomatosis with Polyangiitis

9

Overview

- *Definition*
  - A form of granulomatous vasculitis that affects small- and medium-sized vessels in many organs but most commonly affects the upper respiratory tract and the kidneys
  - Ocular disease can be the presenting or even the only clinically apparent manifestation; can involve any part of the eye
- *Symptoms*
  - Redness
  - Pain
  - Photophobia
  - Blurry vision
  - Diplopia
- *Laterality*
  - Unilateral or bilateral
- *Course*
  - Without treatment, average life expectancy is 5 months
  - With appropriate treatment, long-term remission rate is 93% (lasting from 7 months to 13.2 years); however, half of the patients in remission relapse later in life
- *Age of onset*
  - Fourth to fifth decades of life
- *Gender/race*
  - M = F
  - Caucasian predominance
- *Systemic association*
  - Nonspecific: fever, malaise, weight loss

C. S. Foster et al. (eds.), *Uveitis*, https://doi.org/10.1007/978-3-030-52974-1_9

- Upper respiratory tract: sinus pain, purulent nasal discharge, epistaxis, nasal ulceration, serous otitis media, suppurative otitis, mastoiditis, saddle-nose defect, and hearing loss
- Pulmonary: cough, hemoptysis, dyspnea, pleuritic chest pain, tracheal obstruction
- Renal: proteinuria, hematuria, red blood cell casts, renal insufficiency
- Skin: purpura involving lower extremities or less frequently upper extremities and trunk, ulcers, vesicles, papules, subcutaneous nodules; lesions may or may not be pruritic
- Musculoskeletal: myalgia; polyarticular, symmetrical arthralgia affecting small and medium joints; nondeforming arthritis affecting mainly large joints
- Nervous system: peripheral neuropathies (most commonly mononeuritis multiplex), cranial neuropathies (most commonly cranial nerves II, VI, and VII), external ophthalmoplegia, seizures, cerebritis, stroke syndromes
- Cardiac: pericarditis, myocarditis, arteritis
- Other organs: parotid gland, breast, urethra, cervix, vagina, GI tract

Exam: Ocular

Orbit: from inflammatory mass compression, vascular occlusion, or spread of orbital cellulitis

- Proptosis
- Extraocular motility restriction
- Compressive ischemic optic neuropathy
- Nasolacrimal duct obstruction

Anterior Segment

- Conjunctivitis
- Episcleritis
- Scleritis
- Keratitis
- Uveitis (very rare to have uveitis alone)

Posterior Segment

- Retinal vasculitis
- Retinal hemorrhages
- Vitreous hemorrhages
- Central retinal artery and vein occlusions

- Choroidal infarcts
- Optic disc edema
- Choroidal and retinal detachment

Exam: Systemic

- Upper respiratory: stridor (tracheal or subglottic granulomatous mass)
- Pulmonary: dullness on percussion, diminished breath sounds, crackles
- Musculoskeletal: large joint swelling and tenderness
- Skin: nonspecific and variable manifestations usually affecting the lower limbs, including palpable purpura, ulcers, petechiae, vesicles, pustules, hemorrhagic bullae, and digital necrosis
- Cardiac: pericardial rub
- GI: abdominal tenderness (splanchnic vasculitis)

Laboratory and Radiographic Testing

- ANCA
  - c-ANCA directed against proteinase-3 (PR3) is most specific
  - Some patients may express p-ANCA directed against myeloperoxidase (MPO)
- A low RF titer is seen in many GPA patients.
- ESR and CRP
- CBC
- BUN and creatinine
- Urinalysis
- Chest and sinus X-ray or CT
- Pulmonary function test
- Bronchoscopy
- Lesion biopsy (lung and renal biopsies are most specific)

Differential Diagnosis

- Churg-Strauss syndrome
- Microscopic polyangiitis
- Rheumatoid arthritis
- Infections (*Mycobacterium*, *Nocardia*, fungi)

Treatment

- Cyclophosphamide or rituximab, combined with high-dose corticosteroids in life- or organ-threatening GPA

- Other immunomodulators can be considered for less severe cases, or as maintenance therapy: methotrexate, azathioprine, mycophenolate mofetil, cyclosporine, leflunomide, and IVIg
- Plasmapheresis in rapidly progressive renal disease
- Surgical intervention may be required in orbital disease and necrotizing scleritis
- As it often relapses, lifelong monitoring is crucial

Referral/Co-management

- Rheumatologist
- Nephrologist
- Otolaryngologist

Relapsing Polychondritis

10

Overview

- Definition: Recurrent episodic autoimmune inflammation against collagen types II, IX, and XI, involving cartilages and proteoglycan-rich structures, such as the eye, heart, blood vessels, and inner ear
  - Ocular disease (50–67%): 30% can be the initial presentation of the disease. Most commonly involves the episclera and sclera, but may affect any ocular structure
  - Auricular chondritis (83–95%): unilateral or bilateral auricular pain and swelling; associated with hearing loss, tinnitus, and vertigo from inner ear involvement
  - Nonerosive arthritis (52–85%): asymmetric and often migratory polyarthritis lasting weeks to months
  - Nasal chondritis (33–72%): sudden painful onset with mild epistaxis
  - Laryngotracheal disease (30–67%): varies from asymptomatic to life-threatening complications; hoarseness, aphonia, wheezing, inspiratory stridor, nonproductive coughing, dyspnea
  - Skin/mucosal disease (0–83%): nonspecific and range from aphthous ulcers, nodules on the limbs, to purpura and pustules
  - Cardiovascular disease (6–23%): chest pain, silent MI, arrhythmias, heart block, and syncope from aortitis
  - Neurological disease (0–10%): due to vasculitis of the peripheral nervous system or CNS; peripheral neuropathy, cranial nerve palsy, hemiplegia, and seizures
- Symptoms
  - Pain
  - Redness
  - Photophobia
  - Blurry vision

C. S. Foster et al. (eds.), *Uveitis*, https://doi.org/10.1007/978-3-030-52974-1_10

Table 10.1 McAdam/Michet diagnostic criteria of RP with Damiani-Levine modifications

Recurrent bilateral auricular chondritis
Nonerosive seronegative inflammatory polyarthritis
Nasal chondritis
Ocular inflammation
Respiratory tract chondritis
Cochlear and/or vestibular dysfunction
One of the following is required to establish diagnosis:
≥3 of the above criteria
≥1 of the above criteria with positive histologic confirmation
Chondritis in ≥2 separate anatomic locations with response to steroids and/or dapsone

- Laterality
  - Unilateral or bilateral
- Course
  - Relapsing and remitting
- Age of onset
  - 40–50s but can occur in childhood
- Gender/race
  - Slight female preponderance
  - Equal frequency across races
- Systemic association
  - HLA-DR4 and HLA-DR6
  - A third of cases coexist with other autoimmune diseases, including systemic vasculitis of small, medium, and large vessels; rheumatoid arthritis; ankylosing spondylitis; systemic lupus erythematosus; antiphospholipid syndrome; inflammatory bowel diseases; Behçet's disease ("MAGIC" syndrome: mouth and genital ulcers with inflamed cartilage)
  - RP can also be seen with myelodysplastic syndrome, typically in older males (Table 10.1)

Exam: Ocular

Anterior Segment

- Episcleritis (39%)
- Scleritis (14%)
  - First disease manifestation in 2–3% of RP patients
  - Stronger marker of systemic inflammation
  - Diffuse, nodular, or necrotizing
  - Scleromalacia after repeat scleritis
- Peripheral ulcerative keratitis (PUK)
  - Like scleritis, presence of PUK calls for more aggressive treatment
- Non-granulomatous anterior uveitis
- Conjunctivitis (10%)

Posterior Segment

- Unusual, but retinal vasculitis, vascular occlusion, exudative RD, and inflammatory or ischemic optic neuropathy have been reported

Exam: Systemic

- Auricles: diffusely violaceous and erythematous with sparing of non-cartilaginous ear lobes, +/− sensorineural hearing loss
- Joints: nondeforming and nonerosive arthritis which affect mostly the metacarpophalangeal, proximal interphalangeal joints and knees Sternoclavicular, costochondral, and manubriosternal articulations are also typically involved
- Nose: saddle-nose deformity (17–29%) and a flat nasal tip, more common in men and younger patients
- Large airways: (sub)glottic, laryngeal, or tracheobronchial inflammation with luminal encroachment. Laryngeal collapse during inspiration and/or tracheal collapse during expiration
- Skin: urticaria, angioedema, erythema multiforme, livedo reticularis, panniculitis, and erythema nodosum

Imaging

- FA: retinal vascular occlusion or peripheral vasculitis
- B-scan: sclerochoroidal thickening in areas of posterior scleritis

Laboratory and Radiographic Testing

There is no specific lab test for RP; diagnosis is based on the combination of clinical and radiographic findings, occasionally assisted with cartilage biopsy.

- Labs
  - Elevated CRP is most common, but 1 in 10 patients may have normal acute phase reactants during acute disease flare
  - Serum antibodies to type II collagen: present in 20–50%, but not specific nor sensitive, and only performed in a few laboratories
  - ANA: present in 20–60%; homogenous or speckled pattern
  - ANCA: may be present in RP, but granulomatosis with polyangiitis should be strongly considered if ANCA+, especially if it is c-ANCA and associated with anti-PR3 antibodies
- Imaging
  - Chest radiography: laryngotracheal bronchial wall thickening, airway stenosis, and cartilaginous calcification

Differential Diagnosis

- Granulomatosis with polyangiitis
- Polyarteritis nodosa
- Rheumatoid arthritis

Treatment

- Mild disease with diffuse anterior scleritis and involvement of nasal/auricular cartilages
  - NSAIDs
  - Dapsone
- Severe disease with nodular/necrotizing scleritis and involvement of respiratory tract cartilages, inner ear, and vital organs
  - Corticosteroids
  - Methotrexate
  - Azathioprine
  - Mycophenolate mofetil
  - Leflunomide
  - Cyclosporine A
  - Cyclophosphamide (life-threatening disease with necrotizing scleritis, laryngotracheal involvement, and aortitis)
  - Biologics
    TNF-alpha inhibitors, mainly infliximab, appear effective in many cases after conventional immunosuppressants failed or were poorly tolerated
    Anakinra (anti-IL-1R), tocilizumab (anti-IL-6R), and abatacept (co-stimulatory signaling pathway inhibitor) are effective in fewer reports
    Rituximab (anti-CD20) appears ineffective
  - Plasmapheresis and IVIg used in some cases

Referral/Co-management

- Rheumatology
- ENT
- Pulmonary

Pars Planitis

11

Overview

- Definition
  - A subset of intermediate uveitis that is not associated with a systemic disease or infection and characterized by the presence of snowballs in the vitreous and snowbanks along the inferior pars plana and retinal periphery
  - After idiopathic and JIA, it is the third most common etiology of pediatric uveitis
- Symptoms
  - Floaters
  - Blurry vision
- Laterality
  - >75% bilateral, but can be asymmetric
- Course
  - Gradual onset
  - Chronic with low incidence of remission
- Age of onset
  - Most commonly childhood to adolescence, but also older adults in their 40s
- Gender/race
  - Equal gender distribution in pediatric population; slight female preponderance in older cases
  - Caucasians
- Systemic association
  - By definition, pars planitis is not associated with any systemic disease

C. S. Foster et al. (eds.), *Uveitis*, https://doi.org/10.1007/978-3-030-52974-1_11

Exam: Ocular

Anterior Segment

- Mild to moderate AC inflammation
- Band keratopathy
- Keratic precipitates
- Posterior synechiae
- Peripheral corneal endotheliopathy
- Cataracts

Posterior Segment

- Vitreous haze and cells
- Snowballs/snowbanks (65–98%): must indent sclera inferiorly
- Retinal vasculitis (17–90%)
- Optic nerve leakage (70%)
- CME and ERM common
- Retinal and optic disc neovascularization
- Vasoproliferative tumor
- Retinoschisis (children only)
- Rhegmatogenous/tractional/exudative RD
- Glaucoma requiring surgery is rare

Exam: Systemic

- No systemic findings in true pars planitis, but must keep in mind of DDx (below) and ask pertinent questions

Imaging

- OCT
  - CME
  - ERM
- FA
  - Retinal vasculitis (may be only visible on wide-field FA)
  - Optic nerve leakage
  - Macular leakage

Laboratory and Radiographic Testing

Pars planitis is a diagnosis of exclusion, so systemic diseases must be ruled out:

- Multiple sclerosis: MRI brain/spine, HLA-DR15, and DR2
- Sarcoidosis: ACE, lysozyme, CT chest, Gallium scan
- Syphilis: RPR, FTA-ABS
- Lyme and Bartonella serologies
- Tuberculosis: chest radiograph, PPD, QuantiFERON
- Intraocular lymphoma: MRI brain, diagnostic vitrectomy

Differential Diagnosis

- Multiple sclerosis
- Sarcoidosis
- Syphilis
- Lyme disease
- Cat scratch disease
- Tuberculosis
- Whipple's disease
- Intraocular lymphoma (elderly patients)
- Other conditions that can mimic intermediate uveitis
  - Anterior uveitis with spill-over cells: FHI, HLA-B27
  - Mild vitritis with subtle chorioretinitis: Behcet's, VKH, Eales disease
  - Severe vitritis with visually obscured chorioretinitis: toxoplasmosis, toxocariasis, ARN, endophthalmitis

Treatment

- Treatment is indicated when there is reduced vision, significant vitreous opacities, macular edema, or retinal vasculitis
- Periocular corticosteroid injection (triamcinolone 40 mg/1 ml) with topical steroids if AC inflammation is also present; supplement with oral corticosteroids if necessary
- After three recurrences in the affected eye(s), or in presence of steroid-induced OHTN/glaucoma, or if inflammation is refractory to corticosteroids, treatment should be escalated. Four options:
  1. Peripheral retinal cryopexy or indirect laser photocoagulation to the snowbanks of the inferior pars plana
     - Induces regression of vitreous base neovascularization and consequently stabilizes inflammation

2. Steroid-sparing IMT
   - When disease is bilateral, and/or there is significant retinal vasculitis
   - Anti-metabolites and cyclosporine are first line
   - Biologics including adalimumab, infliximab, and tocilizumab are all effective
     - Keep in mind of association of pars planitis and intermediate uveitis with MS, as TNF-alpha inhibitors – and perhaps tocilizumab as well – can trigger or unmask demyelination
     - Must conduct careful neuro-ROS and inquire about family history of MS and other demyelinating disorders
     - When in doubt, consider neurology consult and MRI
   - Preferred over PPV/cryo/laser (see below) if disease is bilateral or if there is significant retinal vasculitis
3. Pars plana vitrectomy with cryopexy/endolaser
   - When disease is unilateral or asymmetric bilateral, or when there are visually significant vitreous opacities or concurrent VR complications (VH, ERM, TRD)
   - In our experience, this approach alone rarely results in disease quiescence in the presence of retinal vasculitis, but may reduce IMT burden
   - Stronger anti-inflammatory effects than cryopexy/laser photocoagulation along, by way of removing the vitreous which serves as a cytokine scaffold
   - Cryopexy is favored over endolaser in phakic patients to avoid peripheral instrument-crystalline lens touch
4. Fluocinolone acetonide 0.59 mg implant (Retisert)
   - If all else fail, but cataract is a guarantee and glaucoma requiring surgery is likely

Referral/Co-management

- Rheumatology

Multiple Sclerosis

12

Overview

- Definition
  - A chronic demyelinating disease primarily affecting the CNS
  - Episodic reversible neurologic dysfunction
  - Variable clinical course and unpredictable course with four major categories: relapsing-remitting (85%), secondary progressive, primary progressive (10%), and progressive-relapsing (5%)
  - Ocular disease presents as optic neuritis, uveitis, or neuro-ophthalmological disease
  - The majority of patients may show excellent recovery; permanent visual disability is possible if not treated adequately
  - 72% patients with magnetic resonance imaging (MRI) abnormalities convert to multiple sclerosis within 15 years
- Age of onset
  - 30–50 years, but can range from childhood to 60s
- Gender/race
  - F:M = 2:1
  - No racial predilection
- Systemic association
  - Demyelination of the nerves lead to neurological defects affecting the central nervous system
  - Episodic focal neurological defects, paresis and paresthesia may occur
  - Cranial nerve dysfunction is common
  - Difficulty in walking, coordination, and fine motor activity
  - Slurring of speech and difficulty in movements of tongue are common

C. S. Foster et al. (eds.), *Uveitis*, https://doi.org/10.1007/978-3-030-52974-1_12

Optic Neuritis in MS

- Epidemiology
  - In 15–20% of patients, optic neuritis is the presenting feature of their disease
  - 50–75% of patients with MS will develop optic neuritis during their lifetime (usually in relapsing-remitting stage)
- Laterality
  - Usually unilateral, with bilateral cases in 10% of the cases
  - Sequential involvement of both eyes is common
- Symptoms
  - Periorbital or ocular pain that is increased with extraocular movements and usually lasts several days
  - Acute monocular vision loss with great variability
  - Visual field defects such as diffuse loss, central scotoma, arcuate and nasal-step scotomas, and altitudinal defects occur
  - Impaired color vision and contrast sensitivity (>75%)
  - Phosphenes: bright fleeting, flashes of light that tend to be connected to eye movement
  - Uhthoff's phenomenon: worsening of vision provoked by small increases in body temperature attributed to exercise, hot baths or showers, or hot weather conditions
  - Pulfrich's phenomenon: anomalous stereoscopic perception of objects in motion due to asymmetrical conduction between the optic nerves
- Exam findings
  - Relative afferent pupillary defect
  - Optic nerve head may be swollen with peripapillary flame-shaped hemorrhages, and loss of spontaneous pulsations
  - Optic nerve head may appear normal in retrobulbar optic neuritis

Uveitis in MS

- Epidemiology
  - Occurs in 1–3% of MS patients
  - 80–90% of the time presents as intermediate uveitis (anterior uveitis may occur)
  - Third most common cause of intermediate uveitis (after pars planitis and sarcoidosis)
  - No clear pattern in onset between uveitis and MS: one may precede the other and can be separated by many years
  - Incidence is higher in individuals with HLA-DR15 allele
- Laterality
  - Typically bilateral
- Course
  - May be recurrent or chronic

- Symptoms
  - Floaters
  - Decreased vision due to macular edema
- Exam findings
  - AC inflammation (may be granulomatous or non-granulomatous)
  - Vitritis (+/– snowbanking)
  - Retinal periphlebitis (>50%)
  - CME more common in patients with prior optic neuritis
  - Other complications: cataract, glaucoma, ERM, retinal neovascularization, VH, tractional RD

Neuro-ophthalmological Disease in MS

- Oculomotor palsies are common in MS, frequently involving the sixth cranial nerve
- Deficits in pursuit, saccades, and vestibular eye movement
- Ocular flutter, opsoclonus, and saccadic oscillations
- Various types of nystagmus including vertical, vestibular, pendular. Periodic alternating, or convergence-retraction with pupillary light-near dissociation
- Internuclear ophthalmoplegia (INO): limitation of adduction of the ipsilateral eye and rapid nystagmus during abduction of the contralateral eye due to lesions in the medial longitudinal fasciculus
- Miscellaneous: oscillopsia, skew deviation, Charles Bonnet syndrome

Imaging

- FA
  - Optic nerve leakage (except retrobulbar optic neuritis)
  - Peripheral retinal vascular leakage
  - Macular leakage
- OCT
  - ERM
  - CME
  - Optic nerve atrophy from prior optic neuritis
- Visual evoked potential (VEP)
  - Well-preserved wave form but delayed response in 75% of patients

Laboratory and Radiographic Testing

- MRI brain and spine with gadolinium: 3 of the 4 below meet the revised McDonald diagnostic criteria
  - 1 gadolinium-enhancing lesion or 9 T2 hyperintense lesions if enhancing lesions are not present

  - ≥1 infratentorial lesion
  - ≥1 juxtacortical lesion
  - ≥3 periventricular lesions
- Cerebrospinal fluid analysis
  - Elevated IgG index (comparison of IgG levels in CSF and in serum)
  - ≥2 oligocolonal bands via electrophoresis
  - Lymphocyte cell count should be <50/mm^3 and protein should be <100 mg/dL; otherwise seek alternate Dx
- HLA-DR15 can be obtained in patients presenting with intermediate uveitis to assess the risk of MS development (and thus avoiding use of TNF-alpha inhibitors)

Differential Diagnosis

- For neurological manifestations, MS has a board DDx, ranging from ischemic/inflammatory (neurosarcoidosis, disseminated SLE), infectious (Lyme disease, syphilis, PML), toxins (ethambutol), to demyelination (acute transverse myelitis, neuromyelitis optica)
- Other causes of intermediate uveitis with retinal vasculitis
  - Autoimmune: idiopathic (pars planitis), sarcoidosis, inflammatory bowel diseases
  - Infectious: TB, Lyme, syphilis, Whipple's disease, toxocariasis
  - Masquerade: lymphoma

Treatment

- Acute disease exacerbation
  - Intravenous corticosteroids

    Usually first line in cases with acute optic neuritis, uveitis, and neuro-ophthalmological defects

    Accelerates visual recovery in cases with optic neuritis but has no effect on long-term visual outcome
  - Plasmapheresis

    May be indicated in patients with exacerbation of severe, rapidly progressive form of MS and optic neuritis unresponsive to corticosteroids
  - Intravenous immunoglobulins

    Conflicting evidence in cases of optic neuritis
- Treatment algorithm for long-term control
  - In patients with intermediate uveitis, but no neurological symptoms:

    If HLA-DR15 positive, significant retinal periphlebitis on FA, or has a strong family history of demyelinating diseases ➔ refer to neurology for further workup; *be cautious with TNF-alpha inhibitors*

If HLA-DR15 negative, no significant retinal periphlebitis on FA, and no strong family history of demyelinating disease → approach as usual (see above for DDx and see corresponding chapters)

- In patients who present with uveitis, and subsequent confirmed diagnosis of MS:

  Refer to neurology for disease-modifying agents (DMAs), including
  - Injectables: interferon beta-1a/1b, glatiramer acetate
  - Infusions: alemtuzumab, mitoxantrone, ocrelizumab, natalizumab
  - Oral: fingolimod (beware of CME risk), teriflunomide, dimethyl fumarate
  - Off-label: methotrexate, mycophenolate mofetil, azathioprine, cyclophosphamide, rituximab
- In patients with established MS diagnosis but present with a uveitis flare-up:

  Manage the flare-up with a brief course of corticosteroids – topical or regional depending on location of inflammation

  If uveitis remains steroid-dependent or recurs frequently, then coordinate with neurology on choosing a DMA that may be more effective for both CNS and eye (i.e., interferon beta-1a/1b and glatiramer acetate; ocrelizumab should in theory be effective as it is similar to rituximab), or any of the off-label meds as they all are effective in ocular inflammatory diseases

  Avoid TNF-alpha inhibitors, and possibly IL-6 inhibitor (tocilizumab) as well

Referral/Co-management

- Neurology
- Physical medicine and rehabilitation

Lens-Induced Uveitis

13

Overview

- Definition
  - Anterior and intermediate uveitis resulting from a localized inflammatory reaction to crystalline lens proteins
  - Triggering events include
    - Mature or hypermature cataract
    - Retained lens materials after extracapsular cataract surgery
    - Lens capsule rupture following blunt or penetrating trauma
    - Iatrogenic capsular rupture from glaucoma surgery or other intraocular procedures
- Symptoms
  - Blurry vision
  - Photophobia
  - Pain
  - Floaters
- Laterality
  - Usually unilateral
- Course
  - Hours to decades after the causative event
  - Inflammation is persistent and may be severe until lens materials are extracted completely
  - Left untreated, LIU is complicated by severe glaucoma as well as pupillary and cyclitic membrane formation that ultimately results in hypotony, retinal detachment, and phthisis bulbi
- Age of onset
  - 60–70 years

C. S. Foster et al. (eds.), *Uveitis*, https://doi.org/10.1007/978-3-030-52974-1_13

- Gender/race
  - No gender or racial predilection
- Systemic association
  - None

Exam: Ocular

Anterior Segment

- Non-granulomatous or granulomatous inflammation, with abundant cells and flare
- Small KPs (early disease) that coalesce into mutton-fat KPs (late, severe disease)
- Residual lens material in the anterior or posterior chamber (may be visible only on gonioscopy)
- Mature or hypermature cataract
- Ragged or ruptured anterior lens capsule
- Hypopyon or pseudohypopyon (inflammatory cells mixed with lens material)
- Posterior synechiae
- Elevated IOP

Posterior Segment

- Vitritis is always present, though may be obscured by media opacity
- Retinal detachment may occur in severe, untreated cases as the result of cyclitic membrane formation and contraction

Exam: Systemic

- Signs of head or facial trauma

Imaging

- Anterior segment OCT or UBM
  - Useful in detecting retained lens material especially when gonioscopy is obscured by dense AC reaction
- B-scan
  - May reveal retained lens fragments in the posterior segment

Laboratory and Radiographic Testing

- AC or vitreous tap
  - Histologically characterized by zonal inflammation in and around the lens, consisting of lymphocytes, neutrophils, macrophages, epithelioid and giant cells
  - Culture and PCR to exclude infectious masqueraders

Differential Diagnosis

- Sympathetic ophthalmia
  - Bilateral
  - Panuveitis with frequent inflammatory relapses
- Infectious endophthalmitis (exogenous or postoperative)
  - Exogenous
    - Commonly *Staphylococcus epidermidis*
    - Open globe or intraocular foreign body may be present
    - Panuveitis
  - Postoperative
    - Acute: *S. epidermidis*, typically occurring 2–6 weeks postoperatively
    - Chronic: *Propionibacterium acnes*, typically occurring 3 months postoperatively
    - Vitritis is usually mild with a granulomatous anterior uveitis
    - Retained lens material not typically found
- Glaucomatocyclitic crisis (Posner-Schlossman syndrome)
  - Recurrent episodes of elevated IOP, mydriasis, corneal edema and low-grade AC reaction
- IOL-associated uveitis
  - Unlikely with biocompatible, acrylic IOLs
- Uveitis-glaucoma-hyphema (UGH) syndrome
- Consider other causes of anterior/intermediate uveitis if removal of lens material does not result in resolution of inflammation

Treatment

- Steroid, cycloplegic, and glaucoma drops for immediate inflammatory and IOP control
- Surgical removal of retained lens material, either via limbal incision or pars plana vitrectomy, offers definitive cure
  - If retained lens material is minimal and resorption is likely, observation and treatment with topical steroids until all lens material is resorbed may be sufficient

Referral/Co-management

- None

Tubulointerstitial Nephritis and Uveitis Syndrome

14

Overview

- Definition
  - Immune-mediated inflammation involving the kidney and the eye
  - Uveitis is usually bilateral, non-granulomatous anterior uveitis, but posterior segment involvement has been reported
- Symptoms
  - Pain
  - Photophobia
  - Blurry vision
- Laterality
  - Bilateral
- Course
  - Nephritis is self-limited and rarely recurs, but uveitis can become recurrent in 40%
  - In 65% of cases, acute nephritis precedes uveitis by weeks to months; 20% uveitis precedes nephritis; 15% nephritis and uveitis occur concurrently
- Age of onset
  - Children and adolescent, with median age of 15 years
- Gender/race
  - F:M = 3:1
  - No racial predilection
- Systemic association
  - Tubulointerstitial nephritis: injury to renal tubules and interstitium (*not* involving the glomeruli), leading to decreased renal function
  - Several HLA haplotypes have been associated with TINU, but HLA-DRB1*0102 represents the strongest association

C. S. Foster et al. (eds.), *Uveitis*, https://doi.org/10.1007/978-3-030-52974-1_14

Exam: Ocular

Anterior segment

- Non-granulomatous AC inflammation, ranging from mild to severe

Posterior Segment

- Uncommon: papillitis, cystoid macular edema, retinal pigment epithelial detachments, retinal vascular sheathing, vitritis, neuroretinitis, multifocal choroiditis

Exam: Systemic

- Abdominal or flank pain
- Fatigue
- Fever
- Headache
- Anorexia and weight loss
- BP usually normal

Imaging

- OCT
  - CME (rare)
- FA
  - Optic nerve leakage or vascular staining (rare)

Laboratory and Radiographic Testing

- Renal biopsy (for definitive diagnosis): tubulointerstitial nephritis
- Urinalysis: elevated beta-2 microglobulin, mild proteinuria, eosinophilia, pyuria or hematuria without infection, normoglycemic glycosuria, white cell casts
- Bloodwork: elevated serum creatinine or decreased creatinine clearance, anemia, abnormal LFTs, elevated ESR

Differential Diagnosis

Inflammatory diseases that can affect the kidney and the eye:

- Systemic lupus erythematosus
- Sarcoidosis

- Granulomatosis and polyangiitis
- Adamantiades-Behcet's disease
- Sjögren's syndrome
- IgA nephropathy (Berger's disease)
- Post-streptococcal uveitis
- Syphilis
- Leptospirosis
- Brucellosis
- Tuberculosis
- Drug-induced TINU: NSAIDs, Chinese herb *Goreisan*, acetaminophen, codeine phosphate, lamotrigine, smoking synthetic cannabinoid

Treatment

- Nephritis responds favorably to systemic corticosteroids
- Uveitis responds well to topical or regional steroids, but in recurrent cases systemic IMT is employed, including methotrexate, azathioprine, and cyclosporine

Referral/Co-management

- Nephrology

Birdshot Retinochoroidopathy

15

Overview

- Definition:
  - Birdshot retinochoroidopathy (BSRC) is a clinically distinct, uncommon form of posterior uveitis, characterized by vitritis, retinal vasculitis, and multiple, bilateral, hypopigmented, postequatorial inflammatory lesions at the level of RPE and choroid
  - Patient's visual complaints are often out of proportion to the measured visual acuity, and fundus findings can be extremely subtle in early disease stage
- Symptoms
  - Floaters
  - Photophobia
  - Photopsia
  - Glare
  - Some degree of nyctalopia
  - Reduced contrast sensitivity
  - Blue-yellow dyschromatopsia and other color vision disturbances
- Laterality
  - Bilateral
- Course
  - Chronic, characterized by multiple exacerbations and remissions
  - Self-limited in only 20% of cases
- Age of onset
  - 40–50 years
- Gender/race
  - F:M = 3:1
  - Almost exclusively Caucasian, with a higher incidence in those of northern European descent

C. S. Foster et al. (eds.), *Uveitis*, https://doi.org/10.1007/978-3-030-52974-1_15

- Systemic association
  - HLA-A29 association is perhaps most well known in ophthalmology, if not all of medicine
  - Though not as prevalent as HLA-A29, HLA-B44 is found in 50% of BSRC patients
  - Systemic hypertension appears to be more prevalent in BSRC population

Exam: Ocular

Anterior Segment

- Quiet eye without conjunctival injection or ciliary flush
- Mild nongranulomatous anterior uveitis (≤1+ cells) without synechia
- +/− fine keratic precipitates
- Normal IOP

Posterior Segment

- BSRC lesions
  - Multiple, cream-colored, choroidal lesions with indistinct borders, the long axis of which is radial to the optic disc scattered throughout the postequatorial retina
  - Round to ovoid in shape, varying in size from 50 to 1500 μm
  - More easily visualized clustered around the optic disc, in the inferonasal quadrant
  - With time, lesions may become confluent, producing large areas of geographic depigmentation
- Mild-to-moderate vitritis (≤2+ haze)
- Retinal vasculitis (predominantly phlebitis) typically in the absence of visible vascular sheathing
- Retinal arteriolar attenuation and vascular tortuosity may be seen
- CME is the most common structural complication of BSRC (cumulative incidence approaching 84% over 5 years) and is the most frequent cause of reduced central VA
- ERM is common
- CNV and retinal NV leading to NV are relatively rare (<10%)
- Optic nerve head swelling and nerve fiber layer hemorrhages

Imaging

- FA
  - Macular leakage
  - Vasculitis (predominantly phlebitis)
  - Generalized abnormal hyperfluorescence

- ICG
  - Hypofluorescent spots and fuzzy vessels in *active* disease
  - Hypofluorescence often not seen in treated or burn-out disease
  - May or may not correspond to fundus lesions seen on microscopy
- Fundus autofluorescence
  - Abnormal in 80% of patients
  - Peripapillary, macular, or extramacular hypoautofluorescence
- OCT
  - CME and ERM
  - IS/OS attenuation
  - EDI-OCT may show choroidal lesions otherwise not apparent on ophthalmoscopy
- ERG
  - Early (inner retinopathy): loss of oscillatory potentials and b-wave amplitude
  - Late (outer retinopathy): reduction of photopic b-wave amplitude and progressive prolongation of 30 Hz implicit time (IT), used for follow up the effect of treatment
- Blue-on-yellow perimetry (SITA-SWAP)
  - Generalized constriction of the peripheral visual field
  - Central and paracentral scotomata
  - Enlargement of the blind spot
  - Abnormalities on visual field testing may occur even among minimally symptomatic patients with good VA

Laboratory Testing

- HLA-A29 phenotype
  - Present in 7–8% of general population
  - 95–100% of BSRC patients
  - Confers 50–224 times risk of developing BSRC
- Labs to rule out the masqueraders (see below)

Differential Diagnosis

- Sarcoidosis
- Intraocular lymphoma
- VKH
- Tuberculosis
- Syphilis
- POHS
- White dot syndromes: MCP, PIC, MEWDS, APMPPE

Treatment

- Periocular and systemic corticosteroids have inconsistent treatment efficacy and provide only short-term reduction in vitritis and CME, and thus should be used only for acute exacerbations
- A variety of immunomodulatory agents including methotrexate, mycophenolate, cyclosporine, azathioprine, cyclophosphamide, chlorambucil, intravenous immunoglobulin (IVIg), TNF-alpha inhibitors, and anti-IL6 receptor have been employed as part of a steroid-sparing strategy in the treatment of BSRC
- We typically are following this order of therapy in the majority of our BSRC patients:
  1. Combination therapy of mycophenolate mofetil (1–3 g/day) and cyclosporine (100–300 mg/day)
  2. TNF-alpha inhibitors: infliximab 5–10 mg/kg administered every 4 weeks is very effective
  3. Fluocinolone acetonide implant:

     Higher likelihood of concurrent or subsequent glaucoma incisional surgery in BSRC patients

Referral/Comanagement

- Rheumatology

Sympathetic Ophthalmia

16

Overview

- Definition
  - Bilateral granulomatous panuveitis that develops after ocular surgery or penetrating trauma to one eye, causing disruption to the immune privilege of the eye
- Symptoms
  - Redness
  - Photophobia
  - Pain
  - Blurry vision
  - Floaters
- Laterality
  - Bilateral
- Course
  - Average time between injury/surgery to onset of SO: 2 weeks to 3 months (range: 5 days to 66 years).

    90% of cases manifest within 12 months of insult.
  - Onset can be insidious in the sympathizing, noninjured eye.
  - Severity of inflammation and its sequelae are wide-ranging, and relapsing nature of SO requires long-term monitoring.
  - 75% of patients retain ≥20/200.
- Age of onset
  - All ages affected
- Gender/race
  - Males more affected, likely due to higher risk of ocular injury
  - No racial predisposition

C. S. Foster et al. (eds.), *Uveitis*, https://doi.org/10.1007/978-3-030-52974-1_16

- Systemic association
  - Patients with SO are more likely to express HLA-DR4, HLA-DQw3, HLA-DRw53 (also seen in VKH).
  - VKH-like integumentary changes (poliosis and vitiligo) have been reported, but very uncommon.

Exam: Ocular

Anterior Segment

- Mild-to-severe anterior uveitis with mutton-fat precipitates.
- Corneal endothelium may decompensate with chronic inflammation → bullous keratopathy.
- Posterior synechiae.
- Secondary cataract is common.

Posterior Segment

- Mild-to-moderate vitritis
- Dalen-Fuchs nodules: multiple yellowish-white choroidal lesions in the periphery (also seen in VKH and sarcoidosis)
- Diffuse choroiditis
- Papillitis
- Exudative RD
- Subretinal fibrosis
- Retinochoroidal and optic atrophy

Exam: Systemic (Uncommon)

- Vitiligo
- Hearing dysfunction

Imaging

- OCT
  - Varied disruptions of the outer retinal segments
  - Subretinal fluid corresponding to exudative RD
  - Intraretinal edema and thickening
  - Diffuse choroidal thickening best seen on EDI-OCT: may be used to monitor disease and treatment response

- FA
  - Multiple hyperfluorescent leakage at the level of RPE during the venous phase that persist into the late phase
  - Dye pooling in subretinal spaces in severe cases
  - Areas of early blocked fluorescence corresponding to Dalen-Fuchs nodules
- ICG
  - Multiple hypofluorescent foci that become more prominent as angiography progresses
- B-scan
  - Marked choroidal thickening

Laboratory and Radiographic Testing

- HLA typing may help confirm diagnosis.
- Labs are done to rule out DDx:
  - ACE/lysozyme
  - PPD or QuantiFERON-Gold
  - FTA-ABS/RPR

Differential Diagnosis

- VKH (Table 16.1)
- Sarcoidosis
- Syphilis
- Tuberculosis
- Intraocular lymphoma

Table 16.1 Comparison of sympathetic ophthalmia (SO) and Vogt-Konayagi-Harada syndrome (VKH)

Characteristics	SO	VKH
Age	All ages	20–50 years
Racial predisposition	None	Asia and black
Penetrating injury	Always present	Absent
Skin changes	Uncommon	Common (60–90%)
CNS findings	Uncommon	Common (85%)
Hearing dysfunction	Uncommon	Common (75%)
Optic nerve inflammation	Occasional	Frequent
Exudative RD	Rare	Frequent
Choriocapillaris involvement	Usually absent	Frequent
CSF findings	Usually normal	Pleocytosis (84%)

Treatment

- Corticosteroids – both systemic and local – should be instituted as soon as possible.
- Steroid-sparing IMT should be started at time of diagnosis, as inflammation is certain to relapse upon steroid discontinuation.
  - Cyclosporine, azathioprine, mycophenolate mofetil, chlorambucil, cyclophosphamide, and infliximab have all shown efficacy.
- Fluocinolone acetonide (Retisert), if IMT not effective or not tolerated.
- Enucleation may lower chance of SO if done within 2 weeks of open globe injury; ineffective after development of autoimmune inflammation.

Referral/Comanagement

- Rheumatology

17 Vogt-Koyanagi-Harada Syndrome

Overview

- *Definition*
  - Also known as uveomeningitic or uveomeningoencephalic syndrome.
  - Systemic autoimmune disease affecting pigmented (melanin-containing) tissues in multiple organ systems including ocular, auditory, nervous, and integumentary.
  - Eye disease may occur alone or with extraocular manifestations.

    Complete VKH – revised criteria 1–5

    Incomplete VKH – revised criteria 1–3, 4 or 5

    Harada's disease/Probable VKH – revised criteria 1–3
    - Ocular disease only

    Revised criteria
    - No history of penetrating ocular trauma or surgery prior to onset of uveitis
    - No clinical or lab evidence of other ocular disease
    - Bilateral
    - Neurologic/auditory findings
    - Integumentary findings (found after all other findings)
- Symptoms:
  - Blurring
  - Pain
  - Redness
  - Photophobia
  - Floaters
- Laterality
  - Bilateral.
  - Second eye may be delayed by 1–3 days.

C. S. Foster et al. (eds.), *Uveitis*, https://doi.org/10.1007/978-3-030-52974-1_17

- Course
  - Multiple phases
    - Early (prodromal, acute uveitic)
    - Late (convalescent, chronic recurrent)
- Age of onset
  - Typically 20–50 years, may occur in children
- Gender/race
  - Females slightly more than males
  - Found worldwide, more frequent in darkly pigmented races
    - Common in Asian, Hispanic, Middle Eastern, Native American
- Systemic association:
  - Neurologic
  - Auditory
  - Dermatologic

Exam: Ocular

- Early phase (prodromal, acute uveitic) (days to weeks)
  - Early systemic findings days prior to uveitis onset (prodromal phase)
  - Acute choroidal infiltrate or thickening (acute uveitic phase)
    - Early onset exudative retinal detachment
    - Annular ciliary edema or detachment (leading to narrow angle glaucoma)
    - Optic disc edema or hyperemia
  - Vitritis
  - Dalen-Fuchs nodules
    - Collection of mononuclear inflammatory cells
    - Present in *all phases* of disease
  - No anterior uveitis
- Late phase (convalescent, chronic recurrent) (months to years)
  - Granulomatous anterior uveitis
    - Mutton-fat KP and iris nodules
    - Iris atrophy
  - Sugiura's sign – perilimbal vitiligo (most often in Japanese, 85%)
  - Sunset glow fundus – depigmentation of choroid (common in Asians)
    - 2–3 months after acute uveitic phase
  - Foci of RPE hyperpigmentation and atrophy (most often in Hispanics)
  - Posterior uveitis recurrence uncommon
  - Secondary complications occur mostly later in this stage
    - Cataract
    - Glaucoma
    - Hypotony
    - Retinal neovascularization
    - Subretinal fibrosis or neovascular membrane

Exam: Systemic

- Prodromal phase (2–3 days)
  - Sensitivity to touch of hair, skin (72%)
  - Flu-like symptoms including fever, headache
  - Tinnitus (75%, often with ocular involvement)
  - More common
    Dysacusia, confusion, nausea, meningismus, orbital pain
  - Less common
    Vertigo, ataxia, cranial neuropathies, hemiparesis, aphasia, transverse myelitis, ganglionitis
- Acute uveitic phase (weeks)
  - May include signs from prodromal phase
  - Uveitis as above
- Convalescent phase (months)
  - May include signs from prodromal phase
  - Alopecia
  - Poliosis
  - Vitiligo – head, periocular, trunk
- Chronic recurrent (years)
  - May include signs from prodromal phase
  - Uveitis as above

Imaging

- OCT: exudative retinal detachment, intraretinal cysts
- FA:
  - Early (acute) phase:
    "Starry sky" appearance – Multiple punctate hyperfluorescent dots in areas of exudative retinal detachment
    Disc leakage (70–90% in acute phase)
    Choroidal hypofluorescence (delayed filling)
  - Late phase:
    "Moth-eaten" or "salt and pepper" appearance
    - Alternating hyper- and hypofluorescence from RPE window defects and RPE hyperplasia

    Retinal vasculitis
- ICG: early dark background; later choroidal stromal vessel hyperlucence and leakage, hypolucent dots, disc hyperlucence
- B-scan: diffuse thickening of posterior choroid with low to medium reflectivity, posterior pole or inferior serous retinal detachment, vitreous opacities without posterior vitreous detachment, posterior thickening of sclera or episclera
- ERG: decreased amplitudes and prolonged implicit times of all full-field scotopic and photopic responses, usually improves with therapy

Laboratory and Radiographic Testing

- No confirmatory laboratory testing:
  - Rule out other infectious or noninfectious entities, systemic disease
  - HLA-DRB1*0405 association, not definitive
  - Antiretinal antibodies found in 50% against recoverin, carbonic anhydrase II, α-enolase (not felt to influence outcome)
- MRI – differentiates posterior scleritis from choroidal thickening in VKH, detects subclinical ocular or CNS inflammation.
- Lumbar puncture – CSF pleocytosis within 1 week, resolved by 8 weeks
  - Mostly lymphocytes, also melanin-laden macrophages

Differential Diagnosis

- Sarcoidosis
- Sympathetic ophthalmia (will have history of ocular trauma or surgery)
- Primary intraocular lymphoma
- White dot syndromes: APMPPE, MEWDS
- Bilateral diffuse melanocytic hyperplasia
- Lupus choroidopathy
- Uveal effusion syndrome
- Chronic myeloid leukemia
- Posterior scleritis
- Other causes of exudative detachment
  - Toxemia of pregnancy
  - Renal disease
  - Hypoprotenemia

Treatment

- Early phase
  - Early high-dose oral or IV corticosteroids with slow taper
  - Early initiation of immunomodulatory therapy (IMT) associated with better Va outcomes
- Late phase
  - Topical corticosteroid for anterior uveitis flares *without* active posterior inflammation
  - High-dose oral or IV corticosteroids with taper for posterior disease
  - Initiation of immunomodulatory therapy
- Immunomodulatory therapy
  - Antimetabolites
    - Methotrexate, azathioprine, mycophenolate
  - Calcineurin inhibitors (alone or supplemental)

    Cyclosporine, tacrolimus
  - Biologics
    TNFα inhibitors – adalimumab, infliximab
    Anti-IL6 – tocilizumab
  - Alkylating agents
    Chlorambucil or cyclophosphamide
  - Other agents
    IV-Ig
    Subcutaneous corticotropin gel
- Intravitreal therapy
  - Anti-VEGF
  - Corticosteroid injections, implants (isolated ocular disease)

Referral/Comanagement

- Neurology
- ENT
- Dermatology

Multifocal Choroiditis and Panuveitis

18

Overview

- Definition:
  - Inflammatory multifocal chorioretinal disorder of unknown etiology, featuring prominent intraocular inflammation, affecting young, healthy, myopic women
  - Likely on same disease spectrum with punctate inner choroidopathy (PIC)
- Symptoms:
  - Blurry vision with a wide range of visual acuity
  - Scotoma
  - Enlarged blind spot
  - Photopsia
  - Floaters
- Laterality
  - Bilateral but asymmetric, with one eye possibly being completely quiescent and asymptomatic
- Course
  - Chronic and can persist for years
  - Multiple recurrences in one or both eyes
  - Approximately ¾ of patients suffer permanent visual loss
- Age of onset
  - Mid-30s (range 9–69)
- Gender/race
  - F:M = 3:1
  - No racial predilection
- Systemic association:
  - Affected individuals are usually healthy

C. S. Foster et al. (eds.), *Uveitis*, https://doi.org/10.1007/978-3-030-52974-1_18

Exam: Ocular

Anterior Segment

- Mild-to-moderate AC reaction
- Nongranulomatous keratic precipitates
- Posterior synechiae
- Cataracts

Posterior Segment

- Multiple round to oval, yellow-gray lesions at the level of the RPE
  - Size: 50–350 μm
  - Number: several to more than 100
  - Location: posterior pole and midperiphery, with a propensity for peripapillary region and nasal midperiphery/periphery
  - Distribution: singular, clusters, or streak parallel to the ora serrata (as seen in POHS)
  - Inactive scars are round and variably pigmented
- Moderate-to-severe vitritis
- Optic nerve inflammation
- CME
- CNV is the most serious threat to vision; occurs in around 40% of patients and can be subfoveal, juxtafoveal, extrafoveal, or peripapillary

Exam: Systemic

- Inquire about sarcoidosis symptoms

Imaging

- OCT
  - Macular lesions; abnormalities in IS/OS junction peripapillary retinal photoreceptor segments; choroidal hyperreflectivity
- FA
  - Active lesions: early hypofluorescence followed by gradual staining and late leakage
  - Inactive lesions: window defects with early hyperfluorescence that fades later
  - Late disc leakage
  - Macular leakage

- CNV: early hyperfluorescence with late leakage; may be surrounded by a ring of hypofluorescence secondary to RPE hyperplasia
- ICG
  - Hypofluorescence of the choroidal lesions likely represents inflammatory cells and debris at the level of choriocapillaries blocking dye transmission, rather than perfusion abnormality
  - Hypofluorescence around the optic nerve correlates with enlarged blindspot
- ERG
  - Commonly affected and may not recover fully even after disease control
  - Suggests that MCP is more widespread than its clinical appearance
- Perimetry
  - Blindspot enlargement *not* attributed to disc swelling or peripapillary scarring

Laboratory and Radiographic Testing

None specific to MCP, but done to rule out masqueraders

- Chest radiography
- ACE/lysozyme
- FTA-ABS/RPR
- PPD/QuantiFERON-TB Gold

Differential Diagnosis

- Sarcoidosis
  - Must be excluded for the diagnosis of MCP to be made
- PIC
  - Smaller lesions that rarely extend beyond posterior pole expand
  - Usually self-limited with rare recurrence
  - New lesions rarely appear
  - No AC or vitreous cells
  - Normal ERG
  - Even more frequent CNV but less cataract, CME, and ERM
- Birdshot retinochoroidopathy
  - Older patients
  - HLA-A29+
  - Optic neuropathy and CME are frequent, while CNV is rare
- MEWDS
  - Unilateral
  - Rarely produces permanent fundoscopic or visual changes
- SFU
  - Lesions limited to the posterior pole
  - Severe subretinal scarring
  - Normal ERG

- POHS
  - Patients of all ages from endemic area
  - No AC or vitreous cells
- APMPPE
  - Viral prodrome
  - Less vitritis and little to no AC reaction
  - Larger lesions that resolve without recurrence
  - HLA-B7 and DR2+
- CNS/intraocular lymphoma
- VKH/Harada's disease
- Syphilis
- TB
- DUSN
- Lyme
- Outer retinal toxoplasmosis
- Viral retinitis
- Septic choroiditis

Treatment

- Systemic and periocular corticosteroids are short-term therapies
- MCP is frequently recalcitrant to steroid therapy, and IMT is often necessary
- Fluocinolone acetonide implant is appropriate in those unable to tolerate IMT
- Vitrectomy alone yields only short-term visual benefits and does not alter the disease course
- CNV is addressed effectively with intravitreal anti-VEGF and/or PDT with verteporfin

Referral/Comanagement

- None

Multiple Evanescent White Dot Syndrome

19

Overview

- Definition
  - Rare acute ocular disorder of unknown etiology
  - Findings on exam and testing typically fade with resolution
- Symptoms
  - Floaters
  - Blurring
- Laterality
  - Unilateral
- *Course*
  - Acute, transient
- Age of onset
  - Teenagers and younger adults, mean age 28
- Gender/race
  - F:M = 3:1
  - No racial predilection
- Systemic association
  - None

Exam: Ocular

Anterior Segment

- Sparse anterior chamber cells

C. S. Foster et al. (eds.), *Uveitis*, https://doi.org/10.1007/978-3-030-52974-1_19

Posterior Segment

- Multiple small, round yellow-white lesions, 100–200 μm:
  - Near midperiphery, vascular arcades, and optic nerve with foveal sparing
- Macular orange specks of granularity are characteristic
- Mild disc edema
- Minimal vitreous cells in 50%
- Rarely, retinal splinter hemorrhages and mild venous sheathing

Exam: Systemic

- Prodromal flu-like illness

Imaging

- OCT: focal disruptions in the ellipsoid zone
- FAF: acute stage – hypofluorescent lesions with small (<50 μm) areas in the posterior pole
- FA: patchy or punctate, early hyperfluorescence of white dots, often in wreath-like configuration with late RPE and optic disc staining
- ICG: acute stage – normal AV phase with subsequent hypocyanescent lesions that persist into late phases; more lesions than seen on FA or exam
- VF: blind spot enlargement, cecocentral scotomas common
- ERG: acute stage – mfERG and standard amplitudes significantly decreased
- EOG: prolonged latency and decreased amplitude of P100 complexes

Laboratory and Radiographic Testing

- No lab tests specific to MEWDS
- Rule out other infectious and noninfectious disorders

Differential Diagnosis

- Acute posterior multifocal placoid pigment epitheliopathy (APMPPE)
- Multifocal choroiditis and panuveitis (MCP)
- Punctate inner choroidopathy (PIC)
- Birdshot retinochoroidopathy
- Sarcoidosis
- Syphilis

Treatment

- Self-limited and resolves without treatment

Referral/Comanagement

- None

Acute Posterior Multifocal Placoid Pigment Epitheliopathy

20

Overview

- Definition
  - Choriocapillaritis with secondary ischemia of the overlying RPE and outer retina, manifested as placoid lesions
  - Affects healthy young adults
- Symptoms
  - Rapid vision loss with central and paracentral scotoma
  - Photopsia
- Laterality
  - Typically bilateral but may be asymmetric
  - Possible delay in fellow eye involvement
- Course
  - Self-limited over 2–6 weeks, but new lesions can appear during this time
  - Relatively good prognosis (60% of patients have VA of 20/40 or better), though macular involvement can have significant visual sequelae
  - APMPPE does NOT progress or recur → if so, must consider ampiginous/serpiginous choroiditis (aka relentless placoid chorioretintis) and systemic therapy
- Age of onset
  - 20–30 years
- Gender/race
  - M = F
  - Predominantly Caucasians
- Systemic association
  - 1/3 of patients have preceding flu-like illness

C. S. Foster et al. (eds.), *Uveitis*, https://doi.org/10.1007/978-3-030-52974-1_20

  - Others: Granulomatosis with polyangiitis, sarcoidosis, ulcerative colitis, systemic vasculitis, Lyme, TB, group A strep infection, mumps, recent flu vaccine, and Hepatitis B vaccine
  - Cerebral vasculitis is an infrequent but potentially lethal complication:
    Headaches, confusion, dysarthria (slurred speech), aphasia, numbness, seizure, hemiparesis, ataxia
  - Associated with HLA-B7 and DR2

Exam: Ocular

Anterior Segment

- Little to no AC reaction

Posterior Segment

- Flat, well-circumscribed yellow-white plaque-like lesions in the posterior pole, extending to the equator
  - 1–2 disc diameters
  - May become confluent
  - New lesions can develop adjacent to existing lesions or in unaffected peripheral retina
  - Often resolve after 2–6 weeks and replaced by permanent depigmentation or mottling
- Mild-to-moderate vitritis
- Rare complications
  - Retinal ischemia and neovascularization
  - Optic nerve inflammation
  - Retinal vasculitis
  - Exudative RD
  - Venous stasis retinopathy
- No macular edema unless complicated by CNV (rare)

Exam: Systemic

- Prodrome of headache, fever, malaise, myalgia prior to ocular onset
- If complicated by CNS vasculitis
  - Stroke symptoms (weakness, numbness, slurred speech, etc.)
  - Tremor
  - Hearing loss
  - Poor balance
  - Nuchal rigidity

Imaging

- OCT
  - Hyperreflective RPE of lesions during acute phase; becomes irregular in healed lesions.
  - OCT angiography demonstrates choriocapillaris hypoperfusion during acute phase of disease, supporting the theory that the choroidal vasculature is the primary site of inflammation in APMPPE.
- FA
  - Early blockage and late staining of lesions
  - Ring of choroidal hypofluorescence in active lesions with hyperfluorescence in healed lesions
- ICG
  - Hypocyanescence of both active and healed lesions indicating nonperfusion

Laboratory and Radiographic Testing

- No bloodwork if clinical presentation highly consistent with APMPPE
- MRI brain and lumbar puncture if + neurologic symptoms

Differential Diagnosis

- Viral retinitis
- Choroidal metastasis
- Serpiginous choroiditis (ampiginous choroiditis, relentless placoid chorioretinitis)
- Toxoplasmosis
- Pneumocystis choroiditis
- Other white dot syndromes (MEWDS, MCP, PIC)
- Sarcoidosis
- Vogt-Koyanagi-Harada disease
- Sympathetic ophthalmia

Treatment

- Consider systemic corticosteroids if macula is involved with significant vision loss (worse than 20/60).
- If disease progresses or recurs, then the diagnosis should be revised to ampiginous choroiditis (relentless placoid chorioretinitis) → systemic therapy with corticosteroids and IMT should be employed after ruling out infectious masqueraders (classically TB, but also herpes viruses and syphilis).

Referral/Comanagement

- Neurology if + neurologic symptoms

21 Acute Retinal Pigment Epitheliitis

Overview

- Definition:
  - Rare, idiopathic, self-limited inflammatory condition of the outer retina and retinal pigment epithelium of unknown etiology
  - Also known as Krill's disease
- Symptoms:
  - Painless loss of vision
    - Acuity 20/20 to 20/100
  - Central scotoma, seen on Amsler grid testing
  - Metamorphopsia
- Laterality
  - Unilateral or bilateral
- Course
  - Acute onset of symptoms (days) with resolution over the next few months
- Age of onset
  - 20s to 50s
- Gender/race
  - No gender or racial predilection.
  - 2/3rds of case reports described in male patients.
- Systemic association:
  - Flu-like prodrome 1–2 weeks prior
  - No other systemic association

Exam: Ocular

Anterior Segment

- No signs of inflammation

C. S. Foster et al. (eds.), *Uveitis*, https://doi.org/10.1007/978-3-030-52974-1_21

Posterior Segment

- Fine hyperpigmented stippling of the RPE within the macula surrounded by a hypopigmented halo

Exam: Systemic

- Flu-like prodrome

Imaging

- OCT: Dome-shaped hyperreflective lesion of the photoreceptors and outer retina with disruption of ellipsoid (EZ) and interdigitation (IZ) zones; upward displacement of the external limiting membrane (ELM); lesions normalize with disease resolution starting with ELM, then EZ, then IZ
- FAF: slight increase in hyperfluorescence within the fovea and the areas corresponding to whitish dots (acute lesions) seen on examination
- FA: transmission window defects within lesion without leakage with central blocking lesions corresponding to hyperpigmentation
- ICG: mid-to-late phase hyperfluorescence of the lesion
- VF: decreased threshold sensitivity within central field
- mfERG: depressed central amplitudes

Laboratory and Radiographic Testing

- No contributory testing

Differential Diagnosis

- Multiple evanescent white dot syndrome (MEWDS)
- Acute macular neuroretinopathy (AMN)
- Unilateral acute idiopathic maculopathy (UAIM)
- Solar retinopathy

Treatment

- No treatment necessary, self-limited
- Visual acuity returns to baseline within 2 months in 89%
- Notably, oral steroids have been shown to slow recovery

Referral/Comanagement

- None

22 Serpiginous Choroiditis

Overview

- Definition
  - *Note: This chapter focuses on the autoimmune subtype of serpiginous choroiditis. For tuberculous serpiginous-like choroiditis, refer to Chap. 29*
  - Bilateral inflammatory process involving the retinal pigment epithelium (RPE), the choriocapillaris, and the choroid, leaving behind striking RPE pigmentary changes with wavy margins (serpere = "to creep" in Latin)
  - Synonyms: geographic or helicoid choroidopathy
- Symptoms
  - Blurred vision, metamorphopsia, photopsias, and central or paracentral scotomas
  - Symptoms frequently present unilaterally
- Laterality
  - Bilateral, often with striking asymmetry
- Course
  - Chronic with recurrent exacerbation; progressive without treatment
- Age of onset
  - 30–60 years
- Gender/race
  - No gender predominance; primarily Caucasians
- Systemic association
  - No consistent association with a systemic disease has been identified but may occur in patients with viral meningitis, Crohn's disease, celiac disease, autoimmune thrombocytopenic purpura, sarcoidosis, and PAN
  - HLA-B7 (also in APMPPE)

C. S. Foster et al. (eds.), *Uveitis*, https://doi.org/10.1007/978-3-030-52974-1_22

Exam: Ocular

- *Anterior segment*
  - Little to no AC reaction
- *Posterior segment*
  - Sharply demarcated gray-white or cream-yellow subretinal infiltrates with irregular borders, involving the RPE and choriocapillaris
  - Multiple areas of active disease most frequently seen at the distal edges of inactive scars
  - Lesion tendency for peripapillary area, extending centrifugally in pseudopodial or serpentine pattern, leaving extensive chorioretinal atrophy
  - Mild to no vitritis
  - Rarely, macular or peripheral lesions may present without peripapillary involvement
  - Optic disc involvement is very rare
  - Choroidal neovascularization (CNV) at the edge of the lesion is common, and can lead to lesion expansion without inflammation recurrence

Exam: Systemic

- Good ROS and social history taking to rule out TB

Imaging

- OCT
  - Active lesions show hyperreflective areas in the outer retina with no signs of retinal thickening and intact inner retinal layers; inactive lesions are atrophic with full-thickness retinal loss
- FA
  - Active stage: Early hypofluorescence and late hyperfluorescence at borders of lesions
  - Inactive stage: Mottled hyperfluorescence and late staining of the sclera and fibrous tissue
  - Early hyperfluorescence with late leakage may represent CNV at the edge of lesions
- ICG
  - Subclinical stage (choroidal stage): Hypofluorescent lesions with faint edges and the RPE remains unaffected
  - Active stage (retinal stage): Early hypofluorescence with late leakage or marked hyperfluorescence with evident diffusion in the late stages
  - Subhealing stage: A slight late diffusion
  - Inactive stage: Areas of hypofluorescence with clearly defined margins, which become more marked in the late stages

- Fundus Autofluorescence
  - Hypoautofluorescent areas of regressed disease activity and hyper autofluorescent areas of active disease
  - Very useful in detecting active lesions
- ERG
  - Abnormal in extensive disease
- VF
  - Absolute scotomas (active stage) and relative scotomas (inactive stage) corresponding precisely to visible funduscopic lesions

Laboratory and Radiographic Testing

- PPD, Quantiferon-TB Gold
- FTA-ABS/RPR

Differential Diagnosis

- Tuberculous choroiditis
- Syphilitic placoid choroiditis
- Acute posterior multifocal placoid pigment epitheliopathy
- Multifocal choroiditis and panuveitis
- Acute retinal pigment epitheliitis
- Presumed ocular histoplasmosis syndrome
- Sarcoid choroiditis
- VKH/Harada's disease
- Sympathetic ophthalmia
- Outer-layer retinal toxoplasmosis

Treatment

- Early treatment of active disease with systemic or periocular corticosteroids may be effective but not useful in preventing recurrences or progression of the disease
- Triple agent immunosuppression therapy with prednisone, cyclosporine, and azathioprine may be used with rapid remission of the active disease
- Alkylating agents with cyclophosphamide or chlorambucil is the most effective treatment with long-term remission
- Biologic agents like TNF-α inhibitors can also be used
- In TB-endemic area, antituberculous therapy may be beneficial in patients unresponsive to IMT
- Intravitreal anti-VEGF, focal laser photocoagulation, and photodynamic therapy are used to treat CNV

Referral/Comanagement

- Collaboration with Rheumatology or Oncology if aggressive immunosuppressive medications, especially alkylating agents are used

Subretinal Fibrosis and Uveitis Syndrome

23

Overview

- Definition:
  - Chronic, rare, severe autoimmune posterior uveitis associated with retinal scarring and fibrotic membrane formation from RPE
  - Sometimes thought to be on a spectrum of disease with PIC and MCP
    - Clinical appearance over time is distinct
- Symptoms:
  - Blurred vision
    - Poor prognosis, vision may progress to LP
  - Scotomas
  - Metamorphopsia
  - Photopsias
  - Floaters
  - Fellow eye may be asymptomatic but have involvement
- Laterality
  - Initially unilateral
  - Usually bilateral, may be asymmetric
- Course
  - Acute-onset blurring
  - Progressive loss of vision
- Age of onset
  - Typically under 35 years, but may be any age
- Gender/race
  - Most common in young, myopic females
- Systemic association:
  - No known systemic disease associations

C. S. Foster et al. (eds.), *Uveitis*, https://doi.org/10.1007/978-3-030-52974-1_23

Exam: Ocular

Anterior Segment

- Conjunctival injection, episcleritis, limbal phlyctenules
- Anterior chamber cells
- Posterior synechiae
- Iris atrophy

Posterior Segment

- Vitreous cells occasionally
- Acute retinal findings
  - Multiple fluffy yellow RPE lesions, 50–500 μm in diameter in macula and later midperiphery:
    - Linear patter or in clusters
    - Some lesions fade
  - Optic disc edema
  - CME
  - Serous retinal detachment
  - New flares typically occur in close proximity to existing lesions
- Late retinal findings
  - Punched-out chorioretinal scarring
  - Subretinal fibrotic scars and coalescing placoid lesions
    - Distinctive from other multifocal choroiditis
  - Choroidal neovascular membrane in 50%

Exam: Systemic

- Reports of flu-like prodrome

Imaging

- OCT: subretinal fibrotic scarring; +/− CME
- FA: early hyperfluorescence with late staining, fibrosis shows staining
- ICG: entire lesion hypolucent, area may be larger than visible retinal pathology or in area where no pathology is noted
- VF: scotomas larger than fundus exam of lesions, may involve fixation
- ERG: variable, but generally depressed response; mfERG focal loss

Laboratory and Radiographic Testing

- None, rule out other infectious and autoimmune disorders

Differential Diagnosis

- Other white dot syndromes
  - PIC, MCP, APMPPE, ARPE, serpiginous choroiditis
- Sarcoidosis
- Infections
  - Syphilis, TB, toxoplasmosis, DUSN
- Exudative age-related macular degeneration
- Myopic degeneration

Treatment

- Systemic corticosteroids in acute phase
- Steroid-sparing IMT should be used early, variable response
  - Antimetabolites – methotrexate, azathioprine
  - Biologics – infliximab; rituximab in reports
  - Alkylators – cyclophosphamide
- Laser or anti-VEGF therapy for CNV
- No effective treatment for fibrosis

Referral/Comanagement

- None

Punctate Inner Choroidopathy

24

Overview

- Definition
  - Inflammatory multifocal chorioretinal disorder of unknown etiology affecting mainly young, healthy, myopic women
  - May be a subset of multifocal choroiditis and panuveitis (MCP)
- Symptoms
  - Loss of central acuity
  - Scotoma
  - Photopsia
  - Metamorphopsia
  - Photophobia
- Laterality
  - 80% bilateral, but may be asymmetric
- Course
  - Self-limited over several months
  - Recurrence is less likely compared to MCP
  - New lesions are rare
  - Visual prognosis typically good in absence of CNV and subretinal fibrosis
  - Some cases progress to MCP
- Age of onset
  - Median of 30 years
- Gender/race
  - Predominantly female with varying degree of myopia
  - Caucasian
- Systemic association
  - Affected individuals are usually healthy

C. S. Foster et al. (eds.), *Uveitis*, https://doi.org/10.1007/978-3-030-52974-1_24

Exam: Ocular

Anterior Segment

- No AC reaction

Posterior Segment

- Little to no vitritis
- Small (100–200 μm diameter), discrete, yellowish lesions at inner choroid and RPE:
  - Limited to posterior pole, rarely extend to midperiphery
  - Become atrophic and punched out
  - New lesions are rare
- CNV:
  - Very common (40–75%)
  - Major cause of visual impairment
- CME is uncommon

Exam: Systemic

- None

Imaging

- OCT
  - RPE elevation with sub-RPE collections and compression of photoreceptor IS/OS junctions
- FA
  - Active lesions: early hyperfluorescence followed by variable late staining/leakage
  - Inactive lesions: window defects
- ICG
  - Hypolucent, corresponding to lesions on exam
- ERG
  - Normal
- Visual field/microperimetry
  - Helpful in monitoring for scotomata

Laboratory and Radiographic Testing

None specific to PIC - Rule out masqueraders

- Chest Xray
- ACE/lysozyme
- FTA-ABS/RPR
- PPD/QuantiFERON-TB Gold

Differential Diagnosis

- Multifocal choroiditis and panuveitis (MCP)
  - Chronic/recurrent course
  - More intraocular inflammation
  - Lesions more variable in size and extend beyond posterior pole
  - CME more common
  - ERG often abnormal
- Presume Ocular histoplasmosis syndrome (POHS)
- Multiple evanescent white dot syndrome (MEWDS)
- Acute posterior multifocal placoid pigment epitheliopathy (APMPPE)
- Subretinal fibrosis and uveitis (SFU)
- Sarcoidosis
- Myopic degeneration maculopathy
- Toxoplasmosis
- Lyme disease
- Vogt-Koyanagi-Harada (VKH) syndrome

Treatment

- Systemic and regional corticosteroids if lesion threatens fovea
- IMT in rare, recurrent cases
- CNV can be effectively treated with intravitreal anti-VEGF, PDT/verteporgin +/− intravitreal triamcinolone

Referral/Comanagement

- None

Acute Zonal Occult Outer Retinopathy 25

Overview

- Definition
  - A retinopathy characterized by an acute onset of scotomas and photopsia, along with visual field defects and abnormal ERG that cannot be explained by funduscopic exam alone
- Symptoms
  - Sudden onset of scotomas
  - Photopsia
  - Nyctalopia or hemeralopia
- Laterality
  - More often unilateral on presentation, but 75% become bilateral over time (months to years)
- Course
  - Acute onset with a self-limiting course, but recurs in one third of cases
  - Vision stabilizes over 6 months in 80% of patients
    - 70% with visual acuity 20/40 or better
  - + prognostic factors: No fundus pigmentary changes, bilateral disease, male gender
  - − prognostic factors: vitreous cells, fundus pigmentary changes, female gender
- Age of onset
  - Mid-30s
- Gender/Race
  - F:M = 9:1
  - Caucasian predominance
- Systemic associations
  - 50% of patients report antecedent events
    - Viral illness within days to weeks of ocular symptoms
    - Headaches

C. S. Foster et al. (eds.), *Uveitis*, https://doi.org/10.1007/978-3-030-52974-1_25

Pregnancy
Hep B vaccination and tick bite (single cases)

– 30% of patients have concurrent autoimmune diseases, including hypothyroidism, Hashimoto's thyroiditis, Graves' disease, myasthenia gravis, multiple sclerosis, insulin-dependent diabetes mellitus, CREST syndrome, Addison's disease, Sjögren's syndrome, and Crohn's disease

Exam: Ocular

Anterior Segment

- Normal, except for RAPD if one eye is more affected

Posterior Segment

- Often appears normal initially, with very mild pigmentary changes
- Eventual fundus depigmentation ranges from mild to severe, RP-like
- Attenuated retinal arterioles in affected zones
- Mild vitreous cellularity (higher grade = more diffuse outer retinal damage and worse prognosis)
- CNV is exceedingly rare

Imaging

- ERG
  - Despite being focal by appearance, AZOOR causes a global dysfunction of the cones and RPE. Full-field ERG findings are highly variable and there is no pathognomonic pattern
  - Reduction in amplitude and delay in the implicit time of the A and/or B wave response to photopic white light and/or 30 Hz flicker, loss of the cone component from the response to scotopic dim red light
- VF
  - Blindspot enlargement with or without central scotomas that may correspond with mild depigmentation on fundus examination
  - May mimic central lesions
- FAF
  - Best in delineating disease extent and monitoring for progression
  - Trizonal distribution: (1) normal FAF just outside of the boundary of lesion; (2) speckled hyper-FAF within lesion; (3) central hypo-AF indicative of RPE/choroidal atrophy

- OCT
  - Loss of ellipsoid and outer nuclear layer in acute lesions
  - Thinning of outer and inner nuclear layers in chronic, atrophic lesions
- FA
  - Usually normal, but may highlight mild RPE changes; peripapillary annular depigmentation; retinal arteriolar attenuation within the affected zones; slight peripapillary capillary and/or peripheral perivascular leakage
- ICG
  - Affected zones can be hypofluorescent in both early and late phases

Differential Diagnosis

Normal Fundus

- Retrobulbar optic neuritis
- CNS lesions
- Autoimmune retinopathy
- Acute macular neuroretinopathy (AMN)
- Acute idiopathic blindspot enlargement syndrome (AIBES)
- Ocular migraine

Abnormal Outer Retina and RPE

- Acute annular outer retinopathy (AAOR)
- Serpiginous choroiditis
- Multiple evanescent white dot syndrome (MEWDS)
- Punctate inner choroidopathy (PIC)
- Multifocal choroiditis and panuveitis (MCP)
- Presumed ocular histoplasmosis syndrome (POHS)
- Acute posterior multifocal placoid pigment epitheliopathy (APMPPE)
- Birdshot retinochoroidopathy
- Diffuse unilateral subacute neuroretinitis (DUSN)
- Sectoral retinitis pigmentosa

Treatment

- No proven treatment
- Spontaneous stabilization or improvement of vision may occur within weeks to months
- Systemic corticosteroids and acyclovir/valacyclovir can be trialed if vision loss is progressive

Referral/Comanagement

- None

Syphilis

26

Overview

- Definition
  - Systemic infection caused by the spirochete bacteria *Treponema pallidum*
  - Often transmitted through sexual activity, but may be congenital
  - The "Great Imitator" – may cause morbidity to any of the major body organs and can mimic a great variety of disease
- Symptoms
  - Blurring
  - Redness
  - Pain
  - Light sensitivity
  - Floaters
  - Scotoma
  - Usually present without systemic sign of syphilis
- Laterality
  - Bilateral 44–71%
- Course
  - Progressive
- Age of onset
  - Reproductive age but may present in childhood if congenital infection
- Gender/race
  - M > F; higher rates among men who have sex with men
- Systemic association
  - Multisystemic involvement presenting in stages when untreated
  - Considered neurosyphilis when uveitis is present

C. S. Foster et al. (eds.), *Uveitis*, https://doi.org/10.1007/978-3-030-52974-1_26

Exam: Ocular

- Ocular syphilis may occur at any stage of syphilis

Anterior Segment

- More common
  - Anterior uveitis
    - More commonly present with vitritis than isolated
    - Granulomatous or nongranulomatous
  - Interstitial keratitis
  - Posterior synechiae
  - Iris atrophy
- Less common
  - Lens dislocation
  - Chancre at conjunctiva or eyelid in primary syphilis
  - Iris engorgement – "roseola" – middle third iris involvement (rare)

Posterior Segment

- Chorioretinitis focal/diffuse
  - Most common posterior segment involvement
  - Multifocal typically grayish-yellow lesions:
    - Typically posterior pole or near equator
  - Serous RD, disc edema, vasculitis, and vitritis are occasionally associated signs
  - *Acute syphilitic posterior placoid chorioretinitis (ASPPC)* (rare, but characteristic)
    - One or more large, yellowish, circular, or oval placoid lesions at the level of RPE in or near macular
- Retinitis without choroidal involvement/necrotizing retinitis
- Vasculitis +/− vitritis
- Intermediate uveitis
- Panuveitis
- Neuroretinitis
- Benign tertiary syphilis (Gumma): in choroid and iris (rare)

Exam: Systemic

- *Untreated* syphilis may progress to four stages:
  1. Primary syphilis: *Chancre*
     - Appears ~3 weeks after infection and resolves without treatment ~4 weeks after appearance

   - Painless indurated ulcer at genitalia/mouth/skin/conjunctiva or eyelid
2. Secondary syphilis: *Generalized rash, mucocutaneous lesion, and lymphadenopathy*
   - 4–10 weeks after the initial manifestation
   - Maculopapular rash; prominent on the palms and soles
   - Flu-like symptoms, nausea, hair loss, mouth ulcers, and joint pains
   - Self-resolves in several weeks
3. Latent stage: *No clinical manifestation is detectable*
   - Noncontagious
   - Can last in this stage for entire lifetime
     3.1 Early latent (up to 1 year after initial infection)
     3.2 Late latent (after 1 year)
4. Tertiary syphilis: represents an *obliterative endarteritis*
   - Can appear 10–30 years after infection
   - Risk of severe morbidity and mortality
     4.1 Benign tertiary syphilis (Gumma): in the skin and mucous membranes
     4.2 Cardiovascular syphilis: aortitis, aortic aneurysm, aortic valve insufficiency
     4.3 Late-stage neurosyphilis: general paresis and tabes dorsalis

- Neurosyphilis
  - Can occur at any stage of syphilis
  - Cranial nerve dysfunction, stroke, meningitis, seizure, neuropsychiatric, general paresis, and tabes dorsalis

Imaging

- OCT
  - CME, retinal atrophy
  - ASPPC: subretinal fluid, ellipsoid zone disruption, and hyperreflective granular RPE changes
- FA
  - Nonspecific vasculitis: vascular and disc staining, pericapillary leakage
  - ASPPC: Hypofluorescent central lesion in the early phase with leopard spotting (scattered hypofluorescence) and progressive hyperfluorescence in mid-late phase; late leakage from the optic disc
- ICG
  - ASPPC: hypofluorescence corresponding to the macular lesion in both the early and late phases

Laboratory and Radiographic Testing

- Syphilis testing is warranted in *all patients* with uveitis of unknown etiology (Table 26.1)

Table 26.1 Interpretations of syphilis tests

Nontreponemal	Treponemal assays	Interpretation	Further action
Reactive ≥ 1:8.	Reactive.	Current syphilis infection	Clinical evaluation should be performed to identify signs, symptoms, or past history of infection.
Reactive at 1:1, 1:2, or 1:4.	Reactive.	Current or past infection, or due to serofast condition	
Reactive ≥ 1:8.	Nonreactive.	Inconclusive for infection, biological false positive likely	Clinical evaluation should be performed to identify signs, symptoms, or past history of infection. If recent exposure is suspected, redraw sample in 2–4 weeks.
Reactive at 1:1, 1:2, or 1:4.	Nonreactive.	Syphilis infection unlikely, biological false positive likely	
Weakly reactive, Prozone has been ruled out.	Nonreactive.	Syphilis infection unlikely	
Weakly reactive, Prozone has been ruled out.	Reactive.	Past or potential early syphilis infection	
Nonreactive.	Reactive: False positive of treponemal assays has been ruled out by repeating with different methods.	Past or potential early syphilis infection	If past history of treatment is reported, no further management is needed unless recent exposure suspected → redraw sample in 2–4 weeks.

Adapted from Association of Public Health Laboratories. Suggested Reporting Language for Syphilis Serology Testing. December 2015

- Confirm diagnosis with multiple tests via at least one treponemal-specific *and* nonspecific method:
  1. Nontreponemal tests
     - RPR/VDRL
     - Quantify amount of antibody against *nontreponemal antigens*, such as cardiolipin, which is released by host cells infected by *T. pallidum*
     - "Nonreactive" or "reactive" at dilutions titer (e.g., 1:2, 1:4, 1:32)
     - Titers decrease and become negative after treatment → *use to monitor response to therapy*
     - VDRL false negative 30% in latent syphilis, while FTA-ABS only 1–2%
  2. Treponemal tests
     - FTA-ABS
     - TP-PA/TPHA/MHA-TP
     - Immunoassay (EIA/CIA): Treponemal IgG, IgM
       - Confirmatory test
       - Remains positive for lifetime, regardless of treatment status
       - More sensitive than nonspecific serologic test during latent stage
- Direct detection of pathogen from various bodily fluids

  - Dark-field microscopy
  - PCR
- CSF analysis performed in *every* case of syphilitic uveitis
- HIV checked in *all* syphilis patients
- Reliability of testing
  - False positive
    RPR/VDRL
      - Transient (6 months or less) – malaria, mycobacterial disease, HIV, vaccination
      - Long-lasting (greater than 6 months) – SLE, RA, biliary cirrhosis, old age
    FTA-ABS
      - SLE, RA, biliary cirrhosis, old age
  - False negative
    Latent syphilis, VDRL false negative 30% while only 1–2% in FTA-ABS
    Prozone phenomenon
      - Results in negative or weakly positive nontreponemal test
      - No agglutination occurs due to antibody excess, mostly in primary and secondary syphilis → *dilute and retest*
  - Serofast
    Persistent nontreponemal titer after treatment
    Consider persistent infection (? CNS)/retreating when nontreponemal titers do not decrease fourfold within 6 months after treatment

Differential Diagnosis

- Syphilis should be in the differential diagnosis for every uveitis patient

Treatment

- With uveitis, treat as neurosyphilis, regardless of CSF result
  - Intravenous penicillin G 18–24 million unit per day (3–4 million units IV q4h or continuous infusion) for 10–14 days
  - Alternative – Procaine penicillin 2.4 million units IM once daily plus Probenecid 500 mg orally QID, both for 10–14 days
    Ensure compliance
  - Follow nontreponemal titer q6 months
- Supplemental therapy, when needed
  - IM benzathine penicillin G 2.4 million units weekly up to 3 weeks
    To provide comparable total duration of therapy to late syphilis
- Penicillin-allergic patients
  - Ceftriaxone 2 g daily either IM or IV for 10–14 days (beware cross-reaction)
  - Tetracycline hydrochloride 500 mg PO QID for 30 days

  - Doxycycline 100 mg BID for 14 days
  - Macrolide (clarithromycin)
  - Consider penicillin desensitization
- Jarisch-Herxheimer reaction
  - Hypersensitivity reaction to treponemal antigens, released in large numbers as spirochetes are killed during therapy
  - Usually in the first 24 hours during the initial infusion treatment
  - Fever, myalgia, and headache ± increase ocular inflammation
  - Supportive treatment: antipyretics, NSAID
  - Local and systemic corticosteroid, with severe ocular inflammation

Referral/Comanagement

- Infectious disease

Lyme Disease

27

Overview

- Definition
  - A multisystem disease caused by *Borrelia burgdorferi* sensu *lato*, a group of spirochetes transmitted by Ixodes ticks
  - Characterized by skin, musculoskeletal, neurologic, ocular, and cardiac manifestations
- Symptoms
- Varies widely depending on stages of disease
  - Conjunctivitis: redness
  - Episcleritis: redness, irritation
  - Keratitis: photophobia, blurry vision
  - Intraocular inflammation: photophobia, redness, blurry vision, floaters
  - Optic nerve involvement: visual field and color deficits
  - Orbital inflammation: pain, swelling, diplopia
  - Cranial nerve palsy (CN 4, 5, 6, and 7): diplopia, facial weakness
- Laterality
  - Typically bilateral
- Course
- Applies to both systemic and ocular manifestations
  - Early localized stage: self-limited over 3–4 weeks
  - Early disseminated stage: days to weeks after tick bite
  - Late disseminated stage: months to years after tick bite

    Note: Lyme disease can remain silent for months to years between tick bite and disseminated stages; some patients may never have disseminated disease.

The original version of this chapter was revised. The authorship is changed from "Koushik Tripathy, Aniruddha Agarwal" to "Koushik Tripathy, Aniruddha Agarwal, Miriam Barshak".
A correction to this chapter can be found at https://doi.org/10.1007/978-3-030-52974-1_72

C. S. Foster et al. (eds.), *Uveitis*, https://doi.org/10.1007/978-3-030-52974-1_27

- Age of onset
  - All age groups affected
- Gender/race
  - Slight male predominance
  - More common during warmer months
  - Reported regularly in North America, Europe, and Asia
    - USA: Northeast, Mid-Atlantic, and upper Midwest
    - Europe: More common in Eastern Europe (highest prevalence in Austria and Slovenia)
- Systemic association
  - Early localized stage
    - Erythema migrans (also called erythema chronicum migrans) (70–80%)
      - Average of 7–10 days after tick bite
      - At least 5 cm diameter, and may expand by 1 cm/day (up to 20–30 cm)
    - Fever, malaise, fatigue, myalgia, and arthralgia
  - Early disseminated stage
    - Skin
      - Erythema chronicum migrans
      - Borrelial lymphocytoma (rare in the USA, more common in Europe)
    - Central and peripheral nervous systems (30–40%)
      - Cranial neuropathy
        - Facial nerve is most commonly involved (1/3 of cases are bilateral, which help differentiate from idiopathic Bell's palsy); usually resolves with or without antibiotics, but chance of Lyme arthritis is much higher in untreated patients
      - Motor and sensory radiculopathy
      - Encephalitis/myelitis
    - Cardiac (<5%)
      - AV (atrioventricular) block of different degrees
      - Others: myocarditis, pericarditis
  - Late disseminated stage
    - Joints (80%)
      - Chronic or recurrent mono- or oligoarthritis, with each episode lasting days to months
      - Can affect smaller joints, but general predilection for large joints, especially the knee
      - Often asymmetric
      - May be the only Lyme manifestation in children
    - Neurologic disease
      - Peripheral nervous system: cranial neuropathies, radiculoneuritis
      - Central nervous system: meningitis, encephalomyelitis, benign intracranial hypertension, encephalopathy
    - Acrodermatitis chronica atrophicans
      - Bluish-red lesions found on extremities of older females; eventually wrinkled and atrophic
      - Seen in European cases

Exam: Ocular

As with systemic findings, ocular findings vary with different disease stages, and practically all parts of the eye may be affected:

- Early localized stage
  - Follicular conjunctivitis
  - Episcleritis
- Early disseminated stage
  - Uveitis affecting any segment, but intermediate uveitis with significant vitritis is most common
  - Retinitis and retinal vasculitis
  - Exudative RD (retinal detachment)
  - Optic neuritis/papillitis
  - Neuroretinitis
  - Cranial neuropathy (may affect multiple cranial nerves)
  - Papilledema due to meningitis and increased intracranial pressure
  - Pupillary abnormalities (Horner's syndrome, tonic pupil, mydriasis)
  - Orbital inflammation
- Late disseminated stage
  - Episcleritis
  - Keratitis (bilateral patchy and nebular subepithelial and stromal infiltration)
  - Chronic uveitis

Exam: Systemic

- Skin
  - Erythema chronicum migrans: reddish round rash, which enlarges with central clearing (bull's eye or target lesion), without itching or pain, but may have some warmth. Diameter of at least 5 cm; expands by 1 cm/day up to 20–30 cm
  - Borrelial lymphocytoma (aka lymphadenosis benigna cutis): bluish-red lesions with predilection for earlobes in children and nipples in adults; rare in the USA, more common in Europe
  - Acrodermatitis chronica atrophicans: more often found on extremities of older females, bluish-red lesions that eventually become wrinkled and atrophic; rare in the USA, more common in Europe
- Cardiac: bradycardia
- Joints
  - Asymmetric knee or other joint swelling and erythema
- CNS

  - Facial palsy: 1/3 of Lyme-related facial palsy is bilateral: a crucial distinction from idiopathic Bell's palsy, which tends to be unilateral
  - Multifocal asymmetric weakness
  - Decreased vibratory sensation of the lower distal extremities

Imaging

Due to the varying ocular presentations, there is no specific ocular imaging that would be particularly helpful in differentiating Lyme from other uveitic entities

Laboratory and Radiographic Testing

- ELISA screening for serum Lyme antibodies, with confirmatory Western blot:
  - Both may be negative in the initial 2–4 weeks after infection as it takes time for antibodies to develop

Differential Diagnosis

- Coinfection with *Babesia* and *Anaplasma* should be ruled out in patients with ongoing nonspecific symptoms despite appropriate treatment for Lyme disease, or in the presence of anemia, leukopenia, and or thrombocytopenia
- DDx of erythema migrans:
  - Insect bite hypersensitivity: usually more rapid onset (within hours), shorter duration, and smaller size
  - STARI (Southern tick-associated rash illness following the bite of the Lone Star tick-Amblyomma)
  - Contact dermatitis
  - Bacterial cellulitis
  - Granuloma annulare
  - Hyperkeratotic disorder
- Juvenile idiopathic arthritis.
- Rheumatoid arthritis (symmetric joint involvement; more likely to involve smaller joints than Lyme)
- Systemic lupus erythematosus.

Treatment

- Based on IDSA (Infectious Disease Society of America) guidelines, doxycycline prophylaxis is recommended only if
  - Attached tick is identified as an adult or nymphal *Ixodes scapularis* (deer) tick.

  - Tick is estimated to have been attached for ≥36 hours (based upon how engorged the tick appears or the amount of time since outdoor exposure).
  - Antibiotic can be given within 72 hours of tick removal.
  - Local rate of tick infection with *B. burgdorferi* is ≥20% (known to occur in parts of New England, parts of the mid-Atlantic states, and parts of Minnesota and Wisconsin).
  - Patient can safely take doxycycline (e.g., not pregnant or breastfeeding; not child under 8 years of age).
  - If the person meets ALL of the above criteria, the recommended dose of doxycycline is a single dose of 200 mg for adults and 4 mg/kg, up to a maximum dose of 200 mg, in children ≥8 years.
- Early disease/erythema migrans
  - Doxycycline 100 mg BID for 10–21 days
  - Alternatives: amoxicillin 500 mg TID or cefuroxime 500 mg BID for 14–21 days
- Disseminated disease
  - Doxycycline 100 mg BID for 14–28 days
  - Alternatives: amoxicillin 500 mg TID or cefuroxime 500 mg BID for 14–28 days
- Neurological involvement (including ocular disease involving the posterior segment): may need IV (intravenous) therapy; in Europe, oral antibiotics appear to be as effective as IV therapy for meningitis. In the USA, IV therapy is used more commonly
  - Ceftriaxone 2 g once daily
  - Cefotaxime 2 g Q8H
  - Penicillin G 18–24 MU/day divided Q4H
- Topical corticosteroids for nummular keratitis and anterior uveitis, and oral corticosteroids for posterior segment inflammation, once proper antibiotic has been started

Referral/Comanagement

- Infectious Disease
- Rheumatology
- Dermatology
- Neurology

Bartonella

28

Overview

- Definition
  - Gram-negative, oxidase-negative aerobic bacilli that reside in human RBCs and endothelial cells
    Multiple species exist, 8 of 21 are pathologic to humans
  - *Bartonella henselae* commonly associated with neuroretinitis, cat-scratch disease (CSD), Parinaud's oculoglandular syndrome (POGS)
- Symptoms
  - Decreased vision, 20/25 to 20/200, may be worse
  - Floaters
  - Redness
  - Irritation
- Laterality
  - Mostly unilateral, can be bilateral and asymmetric
- Course
  - Onset of ocular symptoms 1 month after inoculation
  - Typically improves in 2–3 months with treatment
- Age of onset
  - Any age, more common in children and adolescents
- Gender/race
  - Occurs worldwide
- Systemic association
  - Cat-scratch disease
  - Parinaud's oculoglandular syndrome

C. S. Foster et al. (eds.), *Uveitis*, https://doi.org/10.1007/978-3-030-52974-1_28

Exam: Ocular

Anterior Segment

- Follicular conjunctivitis
  - Conjunctival granuloma if primary site of inoculation
- Anterior uveitis
- +/− APD

Posterior Segment

- Vitritis
- Neuroretinitis
  - Optic disc edema, significant
  - Macular star – radial lipid exudates, may be outside macula
  - May resolve in 8–12 weeks
- Focal or multifocal retinitis or choroiditis, mass
  - May be highly vascular and resemble bacillary angiomatosis
- Retinal vasculitis
  - Intraretinal hemorrhages and retinal ischemia
  - Vascular occlusion (BRAO or BRVO)
- Serous macular detachment

Exam: Systemic

- Transmission through cat scratch or bite or open wounds exposed to cat saliva or flea feces
- Systemic findings after inoculation
  - 3–10 days – focal granuloma, small erythematous papule on skin at site of bite/scratch
  - 7–14 days – conjunctival injection, chemosis, and water discharge
  - 2–3 weeks – regional lymphadenopathy, malaise, myalgias, fatigue, low-grade fever (faded skin papule)
- Immunocompromised patients
  - May develop disseminated disease – endocarditis, meningitis, arthritis, osteomyelitis, pneumonia, hepatosplenomegaly

Imaging

- OCT: macular thickening, intraretinal hyperreflective deposits, subretinal fluid, disc thickening
- OCT-A: telangiectasias near disc

- FA: early peripapillary telangiectasias with disc and vascular leakage; late disc leakage
- Perimetry: cecocentral scotoma, paracentral scotoma, enlarged blind spot
- VEP: reduced amplitude and increased latency in affected eye

Laboratory and Radiographic Testing

- Serologic testing, IgG, IgM
  - Indirect fluorescent antibody (IFA)
    88% sensitivity and 94% specificity
  - Enzyme immunoassay (EIA) and Western blot
    86–95% sensitivity and 96% specificity for IgG
    Potential for cross-reactivity between species
  - PCR

Differential Diagnosis

- Toxocariasis
- Tuberculosis
- Syphilis
- Lyme disease
- Sarcoidosis
- Behcet disease
- Rickettsiosis
- Chikungunya
- Systemic hypertension
- Diabetic papillopathy
- Anterior ION
- Papilledema

Treatment

- No consensus on treatment
- May be observed in mild-to-moderate immunocompetent patient
- Doxycycline 100 mg BID PO × 10–14 days in >8 years old
  - May also give erythromycin, TMP-SMX, rifampin, or IM gentamycin
- Severe infection – IV doxycycline and erythromycin with rifampin
- Prednisone with antibiotics, 1 mg/kg/day with taper
- Immunocompromised patients may require treatment up to 4 months
- Conjunctival infections may be treated with combination drops and oral

Referral/Comanagement

- Infectious disease specialist
- Other consults depending on presenting systemic symptoms

Tuberculosis

29

Overview

- Definition
  - An airborne communicable disease caused by *Mycobacterium tuberculosis* and three related mycobacterial species (*M. bovis*, *M. africanum*, and *M. microti*). Ocular tuberculosis (TB) is defined as infection in the eye, around the eye, or on its surface
  - Two billion people are estimated to be latently affected with TB, 95% of whom are in developing countries
  - Ocular disease occurs in 1–2% of patients infected with TB
- Symptoms
  - Highly variable, as it can affect any structure in the eye or around the eye. Symptoms range from very subtle, leading to delay in referral and diagnosis, to severe, sight-threatening complications
- Laterality
  - It can be unilateral or bilateral
- Course
  - Chronic course with an insidious onset
- Age of onset
  - All age groups may be affected
- Gender/race
  - M = F
  - Patients are typically from TB endemic regions (especially Africa and South Asia) and/or of Asian or Indian ethnicity
- Systemic association
  - Ocular TB occurs as a consequence of primary infection, dissemination of systemic infection, or reactivation of latent TB, with host's own immune response and hypersensitivity playing a role in propagating inflammation

C. S. Foster et al. (eds.), *Uveitis*, https://doi.org/10.1007/978-3-030-52974-1_29

Exam: Ocular

Adnexa

- Eyelid granuloma
- Dacryoadenitis
- Nasolacrimal duct obstruction

Anterior segment

- Conjunctivitis and conjunctival phlyctenulosis
- Peripheral keratitis, may be ulcerative
- Scleritis, may be nodular or necrotizing
- Anterior chamber inflammation and synechia

Posterior segment

- Moderate to severe vitritis
- Retinal vasculitis
- Optic disc edema with nerve fiber layer hemorrhages
- Neuroretinitis
- Retinal detachment and subretinal abscess
- Circumscribed choroidal tubercle
- Serpiginous-like/serpiginoid choroiditis (vs. presumed autoimmune serpiginous choroiditis)
  - Younger presentation with average age of 30 (vs. 40–50 years)
  - Moderate to severe anterior chamber (AC) reaction and vitritis (vs. little to none)
  - Unilateral (vs. bilateral)
  - Lesions tend to be multifocal and in both posterior pole and periphery (vs. solitary, mainly posterior pole)
  - Initially sparing juxtapapillary choroid (vs. beginning from juxtapapillary choroid)

Exam: Systemic

- Many patients with ocular TB have latent systemic disease, so there may not be any systemic symptom
- Cough lasting >3 weeks, hemoptysis, chest pain, weight loss, fever, night sweats, chills, loss of appetite
- Extrapulmonary TB occurs via hematogenous dissemination and can affect practically any organ
  - Up to 60% of patients with extrapulmonary TB may have undiagnosed pulmonary disease

  - Miliary TB: affects young children, elderly, and immunocompromised; bone marrow is frequently affected, with anemia, thrombocytopenia, and leukocytosis

Imaging

- OCT
  - Macular thickening, cystoid changes, and epiretinal membrane
- FA
  - Vitreous haze, optic nerve head leakage, retinal vascular leakage or staining, and choroidal inflammation with no or mild early diffuse hyperfluorescence, which evolves into late intense hyperfluorescence
- ICG
  - Hypofluorescent spots in early and late phases if there is choroiditis

Laboratory and Radiographic Testing

- Chest x-ray
- Identification of the organism by culture is the most reliable and definitive diagnostic method, but usually not possible when only ocular disease is present
- Purified protein derivative (PPD): 5 mm or more in immunocompromised, 10 mm or more in immunocompetent, including children, and 15 mm or more in Bacillus Calmette–Guérin (BCG)–vaccinated
  - Cheap and widely available
  - Can help distinguish active vs. latent disease
  - Subjective interpretation, false positive in BCG-vaccinated, and false negative in immunocompromised
- IFN-γ release assays (QuantiFERON-TB Gold)
  - More specific than PPD, not affected by BCG vaccination or other atypical mycobacteria
  - Cannot distinguish active vs. latent disease
  - Costly and not widely available in developing countries
- PCR amplification of ocular fluids
  - Allow for rapid analysis and can help identify drug-resistant strains
- No single test offers high enough sensitivity and specificity to be used alone

Differential Diagnosis

- Sarcoidosis
- Syphilis
- Leprosy
- Vogt-Koyanagi-Harada (VKH) syndrome/Harada's disease

- Sympathetic ophthalmia
- Varicella zoster
- Herpes simplex

Treatment

- In the USA, Centers for Disease Control and Prevention (CDC) suggests starting with RIPE therapy (rifampin, isoniazid, pyrazinamide, ethambutol) for 2 months, then rifampin/isoniazid double therapy is continued for an additional 4–7 months based on subsequent culture result (if obtainable), CXR findings, and HIV status
- Generally, a 9-month treatment is effective for ocular TB
- In case of drug resistance, second-line agents are used: streptomycin, cycloserine, P-aminosalicylic acid, ethionamide, and capremycin are all FDA-approved for TB
- Off-label agents include amikacin, kanamycin, and fourth-generation fluoroquinolones
- Corticosteroids may be used judiciously when there is persistent or even progressive ocular disease despite appropriate anti-TB therapy, as hypersensitivity reaction to TB bacilli plays an important role in ocular inflammation

Referral/Comanagement

- Infectious Disease

Leptospirosis

30

Overview

- Definition
  - One of the most common zoonotic infections in the world, caused by gram-negative helical spirochete *Leptospira interrogans*
  - Infection occurs via direct contact with animal blood or urine (farmers and abattoir workers, veterinarians, laboratory workers), or more commonly via indirect contact with contaminated water (farmers, sewer workers, freshwater swimmers/boaters); there is a higher incidence after heavy rainfall and flooding in temperate and tropical climates
  - Panuveitis is by far the most common ocular presentation
- Symptoms
  - Conjunctival redness
  - Photophobia
  - Blurry vision
  - Floaters
- Laterality
  - More commonly bilateral
- Course
  - Systemic disease presents acutely, typically 2 days to 4 weeks after exposure
  - Uveitis tends to occur in the late immune phase (see below), which can be months after acute systemic illness
- Age of onset
  - Young to middle-age adults
- Gender/race
  - Males are more often affected due to occupational exposures
  - Central and South America, the Caribbean, Southeast Asia, and the Pacific Islands

C. S. Foster et al. (eds.), *Uveitis*, https://doi.org/10.1007/978-3-030-52974-1_30

- Systemic association
  - Extremely wide spectrum of presentations, as the spirochete can invade any organ. Disease severity depends on serovar of the infecting organism and host's immune response
  - In general, leptospirosis is biphasic
    Spirochetemic phase: abrupt headache, fever, vomiting, myalgia following the incubation period of 2–26 days; spirochete is found in blood, cerebrospinal fluid (CSF), and kidneys
    Spirocheturic (immune) phase: recurrence of fever, development of complications, including meningitis, leptospiruria, nerve palsies, jaundice, renal failure, pulmonary hemorrhage, ocular symptoms, etc.; 90% of patients have mild, anicteric disease that gets resolved without treatment; the other 10% can have severe icteric disease with jaundice and azotemia, with up to 30% mortality rate
    Weil's syndrome: a particularly serious presentation of leptospirosis in which jaundice and renal failure occur; the biphasic nature is often obscured by rapid deterioration to multi-organ failure and death

Exam: Ocular

Anterior Segment

- Conjunctival hyperemia and subconjunctival hemorrhage
- Non-granulomatous anterior uveitis with diffuse Keratic Precipitates
- Posterior synechiae
- Hypopyon
- Rapid cataract formation (but may resorb in some cases)

Posterior Segment

- Frequently severe vitritis with large clumps and membranes
  - Vitreous membranes are highly suggestive of diagnosis in the right clinical setting, after toxoplasmosis and infectious endophthalmitis are ruled out
- Non-occlusive periphlebitis
- Papillitis with optic nerve head hyperemia and edema
- Cystoid Macular Edema (CME) is very rare

Exam: Systemic

- Fever
- Jaundice
- Aseptic meningitis
- Respiratory symptoms
- Neuropathy

Imaging

- FA
  - Vascular staining
  - Late optic disc hyperfluorescence

Laboratory and Radiographic Testing

- Testing is imperfect; if there is high clinical suspicion, empiric treatment may be appropriate
- Culture of body fluids (blood and CSF during the first week of infection, and urine after the first week of infection, can remain positive for up to 30 days after symptoms resolve) with Ellinghausen-McCullough-Johnson-Harris (EMJH) medium: growth can take several weeks but can be negative if antibiotics are given prior to collection of samples
- Leptospiral antibody detection (serology) by Enzyme-Linked Immunosorbent Assay (ELISA) antibodies can be found after 5–7 days of illness in naïve patients
  - Background seropositivity in endemic areas makes this strategy challenging for diagnosis of acute infection
  - Paired serum (acute/convalescent samples) are preferred
- Polymerase Chain Reaction (PCR) for leptospiral DNA: test blood during bacteremic phase, CSF, and urine a few days after onset of symptoms, aqueous and vitreous fluids
- Microscopic agglutination test (MAT) is the reference standard for testing and may be requested through the Center for Disease Control and Prevention if ELISA or PCR is positive

Differential Diagnosis

- HLA-B27 uveitis
- Pars planitis
- Behcet's disease
- Eales disease
- Lyme disease
- Tuberculosis

Treatment

- Observation may be appropriate for mild cases
- Doxycycline, azithromycin, or amoxicillin for mild disease
- Intravenous (IV) penicillin, doxycycline, or third-generation cephalosporin (ceftriaxone, cefotaxime) for severe cases; systemic corticosteroid is controversial
- Treatment should be promptly started within the first 4 days of illness

- Doxycycline is preferred when differential diagnosis includes rickettsial infection, which can be clinically similar to leptospirosis
- Because ocular compartments can harbor live leptospira long after acute systemic disease, we recommend systemic antibiotic treatment, along with judicious use of topical and periocular steroids, for uveitis
- Jarisch–Herxheimer reaction can occur following therapy

Prevention

- Vaccination of domestic/farm animals
- Avoiding exposure to stagnant water, rodents, contaminated food
- Prophylactic antibiotics for patients at high risk of exposure (e.g., during outbreaks or flooding in endemic areas): doxycycline—200 mg weekly

Referral/Comanagement

- Infectious disease

Brucellosis

31

Overview

- Definition
  - A zoonotic disease caused by the gram-negative *Brucella* species transmitted to humans from livestock, causing a flu-like illness with potentially lethal complications of endocarditis or neurobrucellosis
    - Reservoirs include cattle, sheep, goats, and pigs
    - High-risk occupations: abattoirs, veterinarians, animal handlers, and microbiology laboratory workers
  - Uveitis (80%) is the most common ocular manifestation, usually occurring during acute brucellosis
- Symptoms
  - Blurry vision
  - Floaters
  - Photopsia
- Laterality
  - Unilateral or bilateral
- Course
  - Ocular disease occurs in chronic brucellosis and typically resolves after an appropriate course of antimicrobial therapy
- Age of onset
  - All age groups
- Gender/race
  - No gender predilection
  - Common in the Mediterranean, Arab gulf, India, Central America and South America, Asia, and sub-Saharan Africa
- Systemic association

The original version of this chapter was revised. The authorship is changed from "Jordan A. Ueberroth" to "Jordan A. Ueberroth, Miriam Barshak". A correction to this chapter can be found at https://doi.org/10.1007/978-3-030-52974-1_72

C. S. Foster et al. (eds.), *Uveitis*, https://doi.org/10.1007/978-3-030-52974-1_31

- Council of State and Territorial Epidemiologists (CSTE) definition: "An illness characterized by acute or insidious onset of fever and one or more of the following: night sweats, arthralgia, headache, fatigue, anorexia, myalgia, weight loss, arthritis/spondylitis, meningitis, or focal organ involvement (endocarditis, orchitis/epididymitis, hepatomegaly, splenomegaly)"
- Acute brucellosis
  - Average incubation: 1–4 weeks (but highly variable, ranging from 5 days to 6 months)
  - Often subclinical with mild flu-like illness with no sequelae
  - Symptomatic disease presents with fever, anorexia, weight loss, headache, arthralgia, and malaise, with focal organ involvements
    - Musculoskeletal: spondylitis and arthritis, especially of the sacroiliac joints and large joints of the lower extremities, osteomyelitis of the vertebrae, tibia, and especially knee
    - Heart: endocarditis (most common cause of death)
    - Central nervous system (CNS): meningoencephalitis (change in mental status, seizure, coma, neurologic deficits, nuchal rigidity)
    - Gastrointestinal (GI): hepatic abscess, hepatomegaly, splenomegaly
    - Genitourinary: orchitis/epididymitis
    - Pulmonary: multiple syndromes
    - Hematologic: cytopenia, disseminated intravascular coagulation
    - Dermatologic: variable morphologies of rashes
- Chronic brucellosis (defined as >1 year of symptoms following diagnosis)
  - Can be persistent localized infection (e.g., bone or eye disease) or relapse following treatment
  - Some patients attribute symptoms to chronic brucellosis without objective evidence of infection

Exam: Ocular

Anterior Segment

- Episcleritis
- Diffuse or nodular scleritis
- Nummular keratitis
- Chronic granulomatous or non-granulomatous iridocyclitis

Posterior Segment

- Multifocal choroiditis, either in geographic pattern or in circumscribed nodules, is most characteristic of posterior segment disease
- Vitritis of varying severity
- Optic disc edema or hyperemia
  - Retrobulbar optic neuritis, chiasmal arachnoiditis

- Cystoid macular edema
- Retinal vasculitis
- Retinitis with edema and hemorrhage
- Exudative retinal detachment

Exam: Systemic

Findings are variable and nonspecific

- Hepatosplenomegaly (most common physical finding), lymphadenopathy
- Right upper quadrant abdominal tenderness
- Knee swelling, sacroiliac tenderness
- New or changing murmur (endocarditis), pericardial rub (pericarditis)
- Nuchal rigidity, Kerning sign, and Brudzinski sign (meningitis)
- Tender, swollen and erythematous scrotum (orchitis)

Imaging

- FA
  - Optic nerve staining or leakage
  - Multiple hyperfluorescent lesions with late leakage
- ICG
  - Multiple hypofluorescent and hyperfluorescent lesions, early
  - Multiple hyperfluorescent spots with associated large areas of hypofluorescence, late
- Visual field
  - Bilateral blind spot enlargement or visual field constriction

Laboratory and Radiographic Testing

- Fluid culture for identification of *Brucella* species (e.g., blood, aqueous, vitreous)
- Standard agglutination test (SAT)—most commonly used
  - "Gold standard" test that uses an antigen derived from *B. abortus* to detect both Immunoglobulin G (IgG) and Immunoglobulin M (IgM) agglutinating antibodies
  - Titers exceeding 1:160 are considered significant for brucellosis in endemic areas (1:80 in non-endemic areas)
  - Interpretation of serologies can be challenging in endemic areas and in patients who have been treated previously
  - This test does not detect antibodies to *B. canis*, which requires *B. canis* serology for diagnosis
- Enzyme-linked immunosorbent assay (ELISA)
  - ELISA and SAT both cross-react with other bacteria

  - ELISA and SAT can both give false-negative results early in infection and in immunocompromised patients
- Polymerase chain reaction (PCR)
- Anterior chamber tap or vitreous tap with Goldmann-Witmer coefficient analysis

Differential Diagnosis

- Tuberculosis
- Syphilis
- Sarcoidosis
- White dot syndromes
- Lyme disease
- Outer retinal toxoplasmosis
- Diffuse unilateral subacute neuroretinitis (DUSN)
- Septic choroiditis
- Viral retinitis
- Presumed ocular histoplasmosis syndrome (POHS)
- Vogt-Koyanagi-Harada (VKH) syndrome
- Sympathetic ophthalmia

Treatment

- Adults and children >8 years
  - Oral doxycycline 2–4 mg/kg/day (maximum 200 mg/day) in two divided doses or oral tetracycline 30–40 mg/kg/day (maximum 2000 mg/day) in four divided doses, *PLUS*
  - Rifampin 15–20 mg/kg/day (max 600–900 mg/day) in one or two divided doses
  - This combination is given for a minimum of 6 weeks
- Pregnancy patients and children <8 years
  - Oral TMP-SMZ (trimethoprim, 10 mg/kg per day, maximum 480 mg/day; and sulfamethoxazole, 50 mg/kg per day, maximum 2400 mg/day) divided in two doses for 4–6 weeks, OR
  - Rifampin with ceftriaxone
  - TMP-SMZ should be avoided during the last week of pregnancy before delivery due to risk for kernicterus
- Cases complicated by endocarditis or meningitis
  - Add streptomycin (20–40 mg/kg per day, maximum 1 g/day divided in two doses) or gentamicin (5 mg/kg per day divided in one–three doses) to the above regimen for the first 2 weeks, then extend the regimen for 4–6 months
  - Surgical intervention for deep-tissue abscesses

- About 10% of patients have relapsing infection despite systemic antimicrobial therapy, due to evasion by intracellular organisms
- Topical and systemic corticosteroids are appropriate once antimicrobial therapy has been commenced

Referral/Co-management

- Infectious disease
- Cardiology
- Neurology

Whipple's Disease

32

Overview

- Definition
  - A chronic bacterial infection caused by *Tropheryma whipplei*
  - Primarily affects the gastrointestinal (GI) tract but may affect other organs, such as lungs, joints, heart, kidney, central nervous system (CNS), and eyes
  - Severe abdominal disease leads to malabsorption and is associated with CNS co-morbidities, and can be potentially fatal
  - Ocular involvement (mainly keratitis, uveitis, and neuro-ophthalmic): 6–8%
  - Well-known yet unexplained propensity in middle-aged, white males
- Symptoms
  - Blurry vision
  - Floaters
- Laterality
  - Unilateral or bilateral
- Course
  - Systemic disease is chronic and relapsing.
  - Ocular disease presents late.
- Age of onset
  - 55 years
- Gender/race
  - M:F = 3:1
  - Caucasian
- Systemic association
  - GI and joint symptoms are most common
    - Weight loss (80–90%)
    - Abdominal pain (50–95%)
    - Diarrhea/steatorrhea (70–85%)
    - Migratory, non-deforming polyarthralgia (70–90%)
      - May precede GI symptoms by months to years

C. S. Foster et al. (eds.), *Uveitis*, https://doi.org/10.1007/978-3-030-52974-1_32

- Other findings
  - Intermittent, low-grade fever
  - Lymphadenopathy
  - Cardiac (endocarditis, pericarditis, Congestive heart failure (CHF))
  - Pulmonary (pleural effusion, pulmonary infiltrates)
  - CNS (dementia, supranuclear ophthalmoplegia, myoclonus, hypothalamic signs)
- Possible association with HLA-B27, HLA-DRβ1*13, and DQβ1*06

Exam: Ocular

Anterior Segment

- Keratitis
- Mutton-fat keratic precipitates (KPs)
- Iris nodules

Posterior Segment

- Vitritis
- Pars plana snowbanks and snowballs
- Cotton-wool spots and retinal hemorrhages
- Vitreous hemorrhage
- Retinitis and choroiditis
- Retrobulbar optic neuritis

Neuro-ophthalmic (Less Common than Ocular, about 10%)

- Gaze palsy
- Nystagmus
- Myoclonus
- Oculomasticatory myorhythmia (OMM)
  - Pathognomonic.
  - Pendular vergent oscillations or smooth vergent nystagmus associated with tongue and mandibular myoclonus.
  - Patients often have gaze paralysis, hypersomnia, and arthralgia without magnetic resonance imaging (MRI) change or GI findings initially.

Exam: Systemic

- Joint swelling and tenderness (more commonly large joints)
- Distended abdomen

- Skin hyperpigmentation and nodules
- Murmurs (pericardial effusion)
- Dullness to chest percussion, diminished breath sounds or pleural rub by stethoscope (pleural effusion)
- Peripheral edema (protein-wasting enteropathy)
- Altered mental status (confusion, memory loss)

Imaging

- n/a

Laboratory and Radiographic Testing

- Gastroscopy with small bowel biopsy is the diagnostic procedure of choice.
  - Light microscopy (LM): clubbed villi and a lamina propria infiltrated with Pas-positive inclusions within and outside of foamy macrophages
  - Electron microscopy (EM): characteristic trilaminar outer cell wall structure ("bacillary bodies")
  - polymerase chain reaction (PCR) (done also on vitreous sample): high sensitivity; based on the nucleotide sequence of *T. whipplei* 16S ribosomal RNA

Differential Diagnosis

- Sarcoidosis
- Behcet's disease
- Collagen vascular diseases
- Amyloidosis
- Lyme disease
- Mycobacterium avium complex (MAC) infection
- Tuberculosis
- Histoplasmosis
- Intraocular lymphoma

Treatment

- Initial treatment for CNS and ocular involvements
  - Intravenous (IV) ceftriaxone 2 g BID=twice daily plus streptomycin 1 g QD × 2 weeks, or
  - IV trimethoprim sulfamethoxazole (TMP-SMX) 960 mg BID × 1–2 weeks, or
  - IV penicillin, 1.2 million units QD=once daily plus streptomycin 1 g QD × 2 weeks
- Maintenance therapy for 1–2 years (<1 year is associated with high relapse rate)

- PO=per os=orally TMP-SMX, 960 mg twice daily +/− rifampin 600 mg QD, or
- PO doxycycline plus hydroxychloroquine

- The most common and serious complication is neurologic relapse, even after apparently successful treatment and systemic improvement.
- Therapeutic and diagnostic vitrectomy for marked vitreous opacities.

Referral/Comanagement

- Infectious disease
- Gastroenterology
- Neurology

Rickettsial Diseases

33

Overview

- Definition
  - A group of diseases transmitted by ticks (less commonly by fleas and lice) infected with rickettsias – pleomorphic, intracellular bacteria that primarily affect the vascular endothelial cells and smooth muscle cells of small and medium vessels
  - Divided into spotted fever and typhus groups
  - Classic triad with mild to severe organ dysfunctions (see "Systemic association")
    - Fever
    - Headache and malaise
    - Rash
  - Rocky Mountain Spotted Fever (RMSF) is the most common rickettsiosis in the United States
    - Pathogen: *Rickettsia rickettsii*
    - Potentially lethal
    - North Carolina, South Carolina, Oklahoma, Tennessee, Arkansas
    - >90% contracted between April and September
  - Other spotted fever rickettsioses in the United States include
    - Rickettsia parkeri rickettsiosis (*R. parkeri*)
    - Pacific Coast tick fever (*R. species 364D*)
    - Rickettsialpox (*R. akari*)

C. S. Foster et al. (eds.), *Uveitis*, https://doi.org/10.1007/978-3-030-52974-1_33

- Symptoms
  - Conjunctival injection
  - Decreased visual acuity
  - Paracentral scotomas
  - Floaters
- Laterality
  - More commonly unilateral
- Course
  - Ocular disease is acute and self-limited.
- Age of onset
  - All age groups affected
- Gender/race
  - No gender or racial predilection
  - Anyone living in endemic areas with exposure to rickettsial reservoirs
- Systemic association
- While RMSF is considered the most potentially severe of all spotted fever rickettsioses, many rickettsial diseases can be complicated by
  - Acute renal failure
  - Respiratory distress syndrome
  - Meningoencephalic syndrome (especially the typhus group)
  - Myocarditis
  - Hepatic failure
  - Fulminant RMSF: in individuals with G6PD deficiency, RMSF can result in severe hemolysis and anemia, with life-threatening complications, within 5 days of disease onset

Exam: Ocular

Anterior Segment

- Most common
  - Conjunctivitis
  - Conjunctival petechiae and hemorrhage
  - Conjunctival nodules
- Less common
  - Mild non-granulomatous anterior chamber (AC) inflammation
  - Keratitis and marginal ulcer
  - Iris nodules

Posterior Segment

- Most common
  - Mild vitritis
  - Retinal vascular involvement in half the patients:

Perivascular white retinal lesions
Subretinal hemorrhage
White-centered hemorrhage
Arterial plaque similar to toxoplasmic Kyrieleis

- Less common
  - Choroidal lesions
  - Macular star
  - Branch retinal artery occlusion (BRAO)
  - Exudative retinal detachment (RD)
  - Anterior ischemic optic neuropathy

Exam: Systemic

- Incubation period varies among different rickettsias, ranging 2–21 days
- Characteristic rash appears 3–5 days after constitutional symptoms, though rash never develops in some cases ("spotless fever")
  - Typical progression: wrists/ankles → palms and soles → forearms, neck, face, axilla, buttocks, and trunk
  - Small, flat pinkish spots (macules) → darker and raised (papules) → papules may develop petechia and merge to form larger hemorrhagic patches (even gangrenous in severe cases)
- Patients with spotted fever rickettsioses *other than RMSF* will have an eschar (dark scab) at the site of the tick or mite bite

Imaging

- Fluoresceine angiogram
  - Early hypofluorescence and late staining of large retinal lesions
  - Vascular leakage
  - Optic nerve staining
  - Blocked fluorescence from retinal hemorrhage
- Indocyanine green angiography
  - Mid-phase hypofluorescent dots if choroidal lesions are present

Laboratory and Radiographic Testing

- Anti-rickettsia immunoglobulin G & M (IgG/IgM) and rickettsia deoxyribonucleic acid (DNA) amplification via polymerase chain reaction (PCR) are offered at commercial laboratories
- Complete blood count (CBC) is nonspecific, but may show
  - Thrombocytopenia
  - Hyponatremia
  - Elevated liver function tests (LFTs)

Differential Diagnosis

- Ehrlichioses (*Ehrlichia chaffeensis* and *Ehrlichia ewingii*)
- Human granulocytic anaplasmosis (*Anaplasma phagocytophilum*)
- Measles
- Dengue fever
- Meningococcemia
- Leptospirosis
- Toxic shock syndrome (*S. aureus*)
- Syphilis

Treatment

- Treat suspicious cases empirically, as serologies can take 1–2 weeks
- Doxycycline is the treatment of choice
- Chloramphenicol 50–75 mg/kg/day in tetracycline allergy
- Fluoroquinolones show efficacy anecdotally; penicillin, cephalosporine, and aminoglycosides are ineffective
- Patient should be afebrile for at least 3 days before antibiotic discontinuation
- Topical tetracycline for conjunctivitis and keratitis
- Topical corticosteroids for anterior uveitis

Referral/Comanagement

- Infectious disease

Leprosy

34

Overview

- Definition
  - A chronic granulomatous bacterial infection caused by *Mycobacterium leprae*, mainly affecting the skin, peripheral nerves, nasal mucosa, and eye
  - Also known as Hansen's disease
  - Infection develops very slowly (can take up to 20 years), and possibly spreads through respiratory droplets, but only after prolonged exposure to untreated individuals; it does not transmit vertically from mother to fetus
  - The three major causes of visual disability are as follows
    - Exposure or neurotrophic keratopathy
    - Chronic iridocyclitis with hypotony
    - Cataract formation
- Symptoms
  - Pain
  - Redness
  - Photophobia
- Laterality
  - Bilateral
- Course
  - Leprosy is highly curable once diagnosis is made and proper therapy is commenced
  - Lepromatous uveitis is typically chronic, with little symptomatology
  - Profound hypotony and phthisis bulbi may ensure if systemic disease and ocular inflammation are not addressed
- Age of onset
  - Two peaks: 10–14 years and 35–44 years

C. S. Foster et al. (eds.), *Uveitis*, https://doi.org/10.1007/978-3-030-52974-1_34

- Gender/race
  - Slight male predominance
  - Very rare in the United States; armadillos are naturally infected in Southern United States
  - Between 200,000 and 250,000 new cases per year worldwide
- Systemic association
  - Skin
    - Hypopigmented or reddish skin lesions that are numb to heat and touch, thus at risk of cuts and ulcers
    - Painless swelling or nodules on the face or earlobes
  - Peripheral nerves
    - Enlarged peripheral nerves that are hard and tender to touch
      - Predilection for ulnar, posterior tibial, and external popliteal nerves
    - Untreated, advanced leprosy results in paralysis of hand and feet
  - Nasal mucosa
    - Epistaxis
    - Saddle-nose deformity

Exam: Ocular

External

- Loss of brow hair or lashes
- Lagophthalmos (facial nerve paralysis)

Anterior Segment

- Exposure or neurotrophic keratopathy
  - Focal enlarged corneal nerves, resembling beads on a string (pathognomonic)
- Iridocyclitis is more often chronic than acute
  - IOP is often low
- "Iris pearls."
  - Pathognomonic
  - Arise deep in the stroma of the iris and are opaque, dense, creamy yellow, and firm (in contrast to Koeppe nodules, which are grayish, semi-translucent, and soft in appearance)
- Diffuse episcleritis/scleritis

Posterior Segment

- "Pearls" in anterior choroid
- Nonspecific hyperpigmentation or hypopigmentation of the RPE
- Focal or disseminated choroiditis (rare)

Exam: Systemic

- Hypopigmented or reddish skin lesions with thickening and numbness to heat and touch
- Hand and feet numbness and paralysis; painless ulcers on soles of feet
- Enlarged nerves that are hard and tender to touch (ulnar, posterior tibial, external popliteal)
- Saddle-nose deformity, epistaxis

Imaging

- N/A

Laboratory and Radiographic Testing

- Diagnosis made primarily on clinical findings
- Skin, earlobe, nerve, or nasal mucosa smear/biopsy for *M. leprae* (acid-fast staining)
- Isolation of *M. leprae* from conjunctival tissue, scleral nodules, aqueous, or iris tissue

Differential Diagnosis

- Chronic granulomatous iridocyclitis
  - Sarcoidosis
  - Lyme disease
  - Syphilis
  - Tuberculosis (TB)
  - Herpesviruses
- Skin lesions can vary widely; some top differentials include:
  - Allergic contact dermatitis
  - Neurofibromatosis
  - Lupus vulgaris (cutaneous TB)
  - Systemic lupus erythematosus
  - Cutaneous sarcoidosis
  - Lichen planus
  - Psoriasis
  - Granuloma annulare
  - Onchocerciasis
  - Leishmaniasis
  - Tinea versicolor
  - Tinea corporis
  - Syphilis

Treatment

- Early treatment of leprosy reduces ocular involvement
- Multi-drug therapy (MDT) is curative after 1–2 years, involving 2 or 3 of the following depending on the form and severity of leprosy
  - Rifampicin
  - Dapsone
  - Clofazimine

Referral/Comanagement

- Infectious disease
- Dermatology

Herpesviruses

35

Herpes Simplex Virus (HSV) and Varicella Zoster Virus (VZV)

Anterior Uveitis

- Epidemiology
  - Average age of onset
    - 40–50 years for HSV
    - 60–70 years for VZV
  - M = F
  - Immunocompetent
- Symptoms
  - Redness
  - Photophobia
  - Pain
  - Blurry vision
- Laterality
  - Almost always unilateral
  - Can be bilateral in patients with atopy and other immune dysfunctions
- Course
  - Acute, but can become chronic if not treated promptly
    - Chronic intraocular inflammation may be due to persistent viral replication or immune response against inactivated viral antigens or damaged self-tissue
- Diagnosis
  - Typically made by characteristic findings and history
  - AC tap for viral PCR can confirm and speciate
- Exam
  - Increased IOP, often as high as 50–60 mmHg (trabeculitis)
  - Corneal edema (endotheliitis)

C. S. Foster et al. (eds.), *Uveitis*, https://doi.org/10.1007/978-3-030-52974-1_35

  - Decreased corneal sensation
  - Mild to severe AC inflammation (hypopyon possible)
  - Diffuse stellate keratic precipitates (KPs) (also seen in toxoplasmosis and FHI), but can also have mutton-fat KPs
  - Diffuse or sectoral iris atrophy (also seen in CMV anterior uveitis)
  - Iris hyperemia
  - Complications: hyphema, glaucoma, posterior synechiae, cataract, hypotony, and, rarely, phthisis bulbi
- HSV: Key points
  - Uveitis and trabeculitis can appear with or without corneal lesions (dendritic epithelial keratitis or disciform stromal keratitis)
  - Check for decreased corneal sensation
  - Iris FA shows intact circulation in atrophic area (vs. no circulation in VZV)
  - Given near-universal exposure and seroconversion by middle age, anti-HSV IgG is only helpful if negative, that is, rule out disease; IgM indicates acute infection
  - Can be complicated by encephalitis in immunocompromised
- VZV: Key points
  - Up to 40% of patients with VZV ophthalmicus may develop anterior uveitis; usually within the first week but may be delayed by weeks to months
  - Uveitis can occur without previous zoster dermatitis (*zoster sine herpete*)
  - Hutchinson's sign: cutaneous vesicles at the side of the tip of the nose; greater likelihood of ocular involvement
- Treatment
  - As it is not always possible distinguish HSV from VZV unless PCR is done on an AC tap, we recommend treating all herpetic anterior uveitis with VZV-specific dose for at least 4 weeks

    Acyclovir 800 mg 5×/day
    Valacyclovir 1 g TID
    Famciclovir 500 mg TID
  - Maintenance therapy

    Acyclovir 800 mg QD-BID
    Valacyclovir 500 mg^{-1} g QD
    Famciclovir 250 mg BID or 500 mg QD
  - Topical steroids are used aggressively once antiviral therapy is on board, as long as there is no concurrent epithelial keratitis (in the case of HSV); often tapered very slowly, and some patients may need low-dose therapy to remain quiescent even with antiviral prophylaxis, for example, 1 gtt QD-QoD
  - Topical cycloplegic for symptomatic relief and prevention of posterior synechiae
  - Caution with prostaglandin in HSV uveitis as it may lead to reactive keratiti-sAcute Retinal Necrosis (ARN)

- Epidemiology
  - Age: bimodal with one peak at age 20 (HSV-2) and another at age 50 (HSV-1 and VZV)
  - M = F
  - Immunocompetent
- Symptoms
  - +/− Pain
  - Redness
  - Photophobia
  - Blurry vision
  - Floaters
  - Visual field defects
- Laterality
  - Starts unilaterally, but becomes bilateral in 35–40% of cases within 6 weeks
- Diagnosis
  - Usually made on clinical findings, but aqueous and vitreous samples for viral PCR and fungal/bacterial culture are appropriate in atypical presentation or if there is no response to anti-viral therapy
- Exam
  - One or more foci of necrotic retina with discrete borders in the peripheral retina; may have macular lesions as well
  - Circumferential spread of retinal necrosis
  - Rapid progression without antiviral therapy
  - Occlusive vasculopathy with arteriolar involvement
  - Prominent vitritis and AC inflammation
  - Optic neuropathy/atrophy (disc edema a common early finding)
  - Scleritis
  - RD is very common, occurring in three-fourths of untreated cases within 6–12 weeks; vitreous traction and PVR further complicate matters
- Differential diagnosis
  - Progressive outer retinal necrosis
  - CMV retinitis
  - Atypical toxoplasmosis
  - Syphilitic retinitis
  - Intraocular lymphoma
  - Leukemia
  - Metastasis
  - Autoimmune retinal vasculitis (sarcoid, Behcet's, etc.)
- Treatment
  - Intravenous (IV) acyclovir 10–15 mg/kg TID for 7–14 days, followed by prolonged oral therapy, is the classic approach

    PO valacyclovir 2 g TID may be equally effective as induction therapy

    IV foscarnet is effective in cases resistant to traditional antiviral

- Intravitreal antiviral is repeated twice weekly until retinitis resolve
  - Foscarnet 2.4 mg
  - Ganciclovir 2 mg
- Oral corticosteroids appropriate if vision loss is significant from optic nerve inflammation, but only after 24–48 h of systemic antiviral
  - Topical corticosteroids safe for AC inflammation
- Prophylactic laser retinopexy if there is clear view
- Pars plana vitrectomy for RD

Progressive Outer Retinal Necrosis (PORN)

- Epidemiology
  - VZV most common: two-thirds of patients have previous or concurrent cutaneous zoster
  - HIV/AIDS (CD4 $\leq$ 50) and profoundly immunocompromised patients
- Symptoms
  - Painless loss of vision often out of proportion to exam findings
    - May be NLP
  - Constricted visual field
  - Redness, irritation, photophobia if positive VZV ophthalmicus
- Laterality
  - 70% bilateral
- Diagnosis
  - Based on clinical history and findings, but vitreous tap can confirm organism
  - FA
    - Late staining of active lesions; window defects in inactive lesions
    - +/− focal vascular occlusion
  - OCT
    - Outer retinal disorganization
    - Inner retinal hyper-reflectivity
    - CME
- Exam
  - Characterized by minimal or no AC or vitreous inflammation (clear view)
  - Multifocal patches of outer retinal whitening that coalesce quickly
    - Affect both posterior pole and periphery
  - 50–70% complicated by RD (rhegmatogenous or exudative)
- Differential Diagnosis
  - Similar to ARN
- Treatment
  - HAART to increase CD4 count
  - Treatment otherwise similar to ARN, though visual prognosis often poor

Non-necrotizing Herpetic Retinopathy

- HSV/VZV can also cause panuveitis in the absence of retinal necrosis, with or without concurrent papillitis or retinal vasculitis
- More like ARN/PORN than anterior uveitis, these cases are often bilateral
- Consider this diagnosis when presumed autoimmune panuveitis or retinal vasculitis fail to respond to systemic IMT

Cytomegalovirus (CMV)

Anterior Uveitis

- Epidemiology
  - Most common ocular manifestation of CMV in the immunocompetent
  - M > F
- Symptoms
  - Redness
  - Photophobia
  - Pain
  - Blurry vision
- Laterality
  - Unilateral
- Course
  - Acute and hypertensive in younger patients (20–50 years)
    - Implicated in Posner-Schlossman syndrome (along with HSV)
  - Chronic in older patients (>50 years)
- Diagnosis
  - Typically made by characteristic findings and history
    - Consider CMV when what otherwise appears to be viral AU does not respond to acyclovir or valacyclovir
  - AC tap for viral PCR
- Exam
  - AC inflammation
    - Little to none in acute form
    - 1–2+ in chronic form
  - Increased IOP
    - Much higher in acute form
  - Diffuse stellate KPs
  - Diffuse or sectoral iris atrophy (not always)
  - Iris heterochromia
  - In contrast to HSV/VZV anterior uveitis

    - Normal corneal sensation is normal
    - No posterior synechiae
  - Complications
    - Glaucomatous optic neuropathy (acute form)
    - Cataract (chronic form)
- Treatment
  - Acute form
    - Valganciclovir 0.15% gel 5×/day
    - Topical corticosteroids or NSAIDs
    - Glaucoma drops for IOP control, but avoid prostaglandin
  - Chronic form
    - PO valganciclovir 900 mg BID for 4–6 weeks, then reduce to 450 mg BID for maintenance
      - Monitor for bone marrow and renal toxicities
    - May discontinue therapy after 1 year of disease quiescence (or if repeat AC tap is negative for CMV)

CMV Retinitis

- Epidemiology
  - Often the initial presentation of systemic CMV infection in immunocompromised patients (CD4 typically <50 cells/mm^3)
  - Occurred in 15–40% of AIDS patients in the pre-HAART era
  - ARN-like presentation has been rarely reported in immunocompetent
- Ocular symptoms
  - May be minimal or absent initially
  - Vision loss
  - Floaters
  - Unspecific visual disturbances
- Laterality
  - Unilateral or bilateral
- Course
  - Slowly progressive retinal necrosis (0.2 mm/week) affecting the posterior pole, the periphery, or both; if untreated, destroy the entire fundus over 3–6 months
- Systemic association
  - Fever
  - Leukopenia
  - Arthralgia
  - Pneumonitis
  - Hepatitis
  - Colitis
  - +CMV in blood and urine

- Diagnosis
  - Typically made by characteristic findings and history
  - Vitreous tap for unclear cases
  - DFE q3–4 months is recommended in patients with CD4 <50 cells/mm
- Exam
  - Little or no AC inflammation
  - Early retinitis may disguise as cotton-wool spots, which is common in HIV retinopathy; however, lesion enlarges with irregular borders and is surrounded by satellite infiltrates
  - Three clinical variants:

    Classic, fulminant hemorrhagic necrotizing retinitis that extends along the major vascular arcades in the posterior pole

    Granular, indolent form more often found in the periphery; little or no retinal edema, fewer hemorrhages, less vascular sheathing, and retinal atrophy

    Perivascular form often described as a variant of frosted branch angiitis, with scattered retinal hemorrhages
  - While primary involvement is rare, optic nerve infiltration can occur if retinitis spread toward the posterior pole
  - Rhegmatogenous RD in one-fourth of patients
- Treatment

  Treatment should be tailored based on the location and severity of the retinitis, as well as host's immune status. UL97 mutation confers treatment resistance in as many as one-third of patients; ensuring HAART compliance and employing combination therapy are crucial
  - Ganciclovir

    Intravenous: 5 mg/kg BID × 2–3 weeks for induction, then QD for maintenance; AE: bone marrow suppression

    Oral: 1 g TID for maintenance (not used for induction)

    Intravitreal: 2 mg twice weekly x 3 weeks for induction, then 2 mg weekly for maintenance

    4.5 mg surgical implant: replaced every 6–8 months
  - Foscarnet

    Intravenous: 60 mg/kg TID × 2–3 weeks for induction, then 90 mg/kg/day for maintenance; AE: nephrotoxicity

    Intravitreal: 2.4 mg twice weekly × 3 weeks for induction, then 2.4 mg weekly for maintenance
  - Cidofovir

    Intravenous 5 mg/kg weekly × 2 weeks for induction, then 3–5 mg/kg q2 weeks for maintenance; AE: nephropathy and hypotony uveitis (co-administering probenecid reduces risk)

    Intravitreal: 20 μg every 5–6 weeks
  - Valganciclovir

    Oral: 900 mg BID × 2–3 weeks for induction, then 900 mg QD for maintenance; AE: bone marrow suppression

Rift Valley Fever

36

Overview

- Definition
  - Epizootic acute febrile illness primarily affecting domesticated sheep and cattle with the capacity to infect humans, caused by Rift Valley fever (RVF) virus, an arthropod-borne phlebovirus in the Bunyaviridae family
  - Transmitted via contact with body fluids of infected livestock or, less commonly, bites by infected mosquitoes. Human-to-human transmission has not been reported
  - Presentation ranges from mild to lethal, with most feared complications being hemorrhagic fever and encephalitis
  - Ocular manifestations are common (1–10%)
- Symptoms
  - Decreased visual acuity and floaters, beginning 1–3 weeks after fever onset
- Laterality
  - Unilateral or bilateral
- Course
  - Ocular lesions are acute and resolve over 2–3 months, though permanent visual loss may occur if macula is involved
- Age of onset
  - No specific age group
- Gender/race
  - No gender or racial predilection
  - Southern and Eastern Africa
- Systemic association
  - Mild cases present with fever, dizziness, headache, back pain, and generalized weakness

C. S. Foster et al. (eds.), *Uveitis*, https://doi.org/10.1007/978-3-030-52974-1_36

  - More severe and potentially lethal cases may lead to seizures or coma due to central nervous system (CNS) involvement and bleeding due to hemorrhagic fever
  - Death occurs in <1% of RVF

Exam: Ocular

Anterior Segment

- Conjunctival injection
- Anterior uveitis

Posterior Segment

- Vitreous cells
- Macular and paramacular exudative-like lesions with retinal edema and hemorrhages have been reported
- Vascular sheathing

Exam: Systemic

- Meningeal signs: neck stiffness, photophobia, confusion, vertigo, convulsions
- Bloody vomitus and stool
- Widespread bleeding involving nose, gums, and skin
- Jaundice

Imaging

- OCT
  - Macular edema
- FA
  - Delayed filling of both retinal and choroidal circulations
  - Macular leakage

Laboratory and Radiographic Testing

- Virus isolation via cell culture, ELISA, or PCR
- Anti-RVF IgG and IgM

Differential Diagnosis

- Measles
- Rubella
- Influenza
- Lyme disease

Treatment

- Supportive care for hemorrhagic and neurologic complications
- No reported treatment for ocular complications
- Vaccination of cattle and sheep is key to prevent the epidemic (no human vaccine available)

Referral/Co-management

- Infectious Disease
- Neurology

Measles (Rubeola)

37

Overview

- Definition
  - Acute, highly contagious, airborne disease caused by Paramyxoviridae ribonucleic acid (RNA) virus
  - While rare in the United States after the measles, mumps, and rubella (MMR) vaccine was introduced in 1965, it is the fifth leading cause of death worldwide in children <5 years of age
- Symptoms
  - Redness
  - Tearing
  - Blurry vision
  - Sudden loss of vision if + retinopathy, after rash
- Laterality
  - Bilateral
- Course
  - Self-limited; visual acuity may be affected by retinopathy initially, but generally recovery over weeks to months
- Age of onset
  - Children and young adolescents
- Gender/race
  - No gender or racial predilection
- Systemic association
  - Congenital measles

    Infection during third trimester results in abortion in 20% of women

    Premature birth common

    Cardiopathy, pyloric stenosis, genu valgum, deafness, mongolism, vertebral anomalies, cleft lip/palate, rudimentary ear

C. S. Foster et al. (eds.), *Uveitis*, https://doi.org/10.1007/978-3-030-52974-1_37

  - Acquired measles
    Generalized rash for 3+ days
    Classic Triad: Cough, coryza, and conjunctivitis
    Possible complications: encephalitis, myocarditis, glomerulonephritis, otitis media, laryngotracheitis, pneumonia, disseminated intravascular coagulation, appendicitis

Exam: Ocular

External

- Dacryostenosis (congenital measles only)

Anterior Segment

- Mild, non-purulent papillary conjunctivitis
  - The most common ocular manifestation along with keratitis
  - +/– pseudomembrane
  - Stimson's line: sharply demarcated transverse injection of lower lid margin
- Epithelial keratitis
  - Begins at limbus and spreads centrally
  - Normal corneal sensation
  - Corneal scarring is cause of "post-measles blindness" worldwide
- Hirschberg spots: Koplik's spots at caruncle
- Cataracts (congenital measles only)

Posterior Segment

- Retinopathy with salt and pepper pattern involving the posterior pole and periphery
  - 1–2 weeks after onset of body rash
- Neuroretinitis (blurry disc margin with possible star-shaped macular edema)
- Attenuated arterioles
- Scattered retinal hemorrhages

Exam: Systemic

- Rash starts as pink macules behind ear, on forehead, and on neck, then rapidly becomes maculopapular and spreads downwards over 3 days to face, trunk, arms, and legs

- Fever >101°F
- Respiratory mucosal inflammation with petechial lesions of palate and pharynx
- Koplik's spots of buccal mucosa (small, bluish-white spots surrounded by a red areola): 1–2 days after rash onset

Imaging

- FA
  - Windows defect from RPE changes
- ERG
  - Normal or mildly reduced response
- Perimetry
  - May be constricted

Laboratory and Radiographic Testing

- Viral culture by swabbing of nasopharynx and conjunctiva

Differential Diagnosis

Congenital Measles

- TORCH infections
  - *T*oxoplasmosis
  - *O*ther infections (syphilis, parvovirus, varicella zoster, Zika)
  - *R*ubella
  - *C*ytomegalovirus
  - *H*erpes simplex

Acquired Measles

- Retinitis pigmentosa
- Toxoplasma retinochoroiditis
- Vogt-Koyanagi-Harada syndrome
- Other causes of neuroretinitis, including Bartonella, Lyme, leptospirosis, toxocariasis, and mumps

Treatment

- No known treatment for congenital form

- For acquired form, gamma-globulin 0.25 mL/kg body weight recommended for high risk patients (pregnant, child <1 year, immunosuppressed)
- Topical NSAIDs and artificial tears to reduce conjunctival hyperemia
- Topical antibiotics to prevent secondary bacterial keratitis
- Systemic corticosteroids for cases of severe retinopathy

Referral/Co-management

- Appropriate specialists for specific systemic complications

Rubella

38

Overview

- Definition
  - An acute, contagious, exanthematous disease caused by Rubrivirus
  - Spread only by humans, via respiratory route or transplacentally
  - Essentially extinct in the United States after the introduction of the measles, mumps, and rubella (MMR) vaccines in 1969; about 20,000 were born with congenital disease in mid-1960s
  - In the United States, acquired cases are typically contracted from foreign visitors or travel
- Symptoms
  - Redness
  - Purulent discharge
  - Photophobia
  - Sudden vision loss
- Laterality
  - Unilateral or bilateral
- Course
  - Acute and self-limited
- Age of onset
  - All age groups affected
- Gender/race
  - No gender or racial predilection
- Systemic association
  - Congenital rubella syndrome (CRS)

    Cardiac, hearing, and ocular defects

    Severity depends on time of maternal disease contraction: most severe during first trimester (miscarriage may result); defects unlikely after 20 weeks gestation

C. S. Foster et al. (eds.), *Uveitis*, https://doi.org/10.1007/978-3-030-52974-1_38

- Acquired rubella (German measles)
  Spread by respiratory route; common in spring and winter
  Incubation period of 2–3 weeks; hosts are contagious 1 week prior to rash onset and throughout active symptoms

Exam: Ocular

Congenital Rubella

Ocular findings can be present at birth, shortly after birth, or later in life

- Salt-and-pepper retinopathy (inactive chorioretinitis, usually confined to RPE)
  - Unilateral or bilateral
  - Typically stable but may progress later in life
  - Vision ranges from normal to 20/200
  - Rarely complicated by CNV. May have focal necrosis of ciliary epithelium, pars plicata, or pars plana
- Nuclear cataract
  - Significant AC inflammation after cataract extraction due to liberation of live virus from lens. Some cataracts have been known to resorb, leaving KP's behind
- Glaucoma
  - Corneal clouding and buphthalmos
- Microphthalmia

Acquired Rubella

- Conjunctivitis
  - Most common ocular finding (70%)
- Epithelial keratitis
  - Infrequent and resolves without sequelae within 1 week
- Retinitis
  - Rare
  - May present as multifocal exudative RD and RPE detachment
  - No retinal hemorrhage
- Chronic rubella has been implicated as a cause of Fuchs' heterochromic iridocyclitis (Chap. 11)

Exam: Systemic

Congenital Rubella

- Unilateral or bilateral deafness (>80%)
- Cardiac malformations: patent ductus arteriosus, peripheral pulmonary artery stenosis, and interventricular septal defects

Acquired Rubella

- Rubella exanthem
  - Erythematous and maculopapular
  - Spreads from face down to hands and feet over 24 hours
  - Resolves by day 3 (thus second nickname "3-day measles")
  - Not always present
- Fever
  - Variable
  - After rash in children; before rash in adolescents and adults
- Postauricular and suboccipital lymphadenopathy
- Other complications: arthritis, encephalitis, thrombocytopenic purpura

Imaging

- FA
  - Abnormal hyperfluorescence and hypofluorescence in salt-and-pepper retinopathy
  - Early hyperfluorescence with late leakage in CNV
  - Hyperfluorescence associated with area of retinitis without vascular leakage in acquired rubella
- ERG
  - Normal in salt-and-pepper retinopathy

Laboratory and Radiographic Testing

- Maternal serum rubella titers
- Viral culture and/or reverse-transcriptase PCR of amniotic fluid, nose, throat, urine, blood, or cerebrospinal fluid (CSF)
- Serum IgM titer is useful in children with anomalies from uneventful pregnancies
- Hearing test
- Echocardiogram

Differential Diagnosis

Congenital Anomalies

- TORCH infections
  - *T*oxoplasmosis
  - *O*ther infections (syphilis, parvovirus, varicella zoster, Zika)
  - *R*ubella
  - *C*ytomegalovirus
  - *H*erpes simplex

Salt-and-pepper Retinopathy

- Congenital syphilis
- Congenital measles
- Leber's congenital amaurosis
- Retinitis pigmentosa carrier
- Choroideremia carrier
- Albinism carrier
- Cystinosis
- Drug toxicity (e.g., phenothiazine)
- Kearns–Sayre syndrome

Salt-and-pepper Retinopathy and Hearing Loss

- Congenital syphilis
- Usher's syndrome

Treatment

Congenital Rubella

- Mothers infected during first trimester should be counseled about possible birth defects
- Immune globulin within 72 hours of exposure during pregnancy
- Rubella vaccination is contraindicated during pregnancy
- CRS infants are contagious at birth and need isolation

Acquired Rubella

- Treatment is supportive, as there is no known antiviral therapy for rubella
- Topical NSAIDs and artificial tears to reduce conjunctival hyperemia
- Retinitis can benefit from corticosteroids

Referral/Co-management

- Audiology
- Cardiology
- Infectious Disease

39 Emergent Viral Infections

- There has been increased awareness of the following viruses and their ophthalmologic comorbidities with the advent of recent elevation in worldwide exposure, including epidemics, after increases in global travel and enterprise
  - West Nile virus (WNV)
  - Dengue virus (DFV)
  - Chikungunya (CHK)
  - Zika virus (ZKV)

West Nile Virus (WNV)

Overview

- Definition
  - Single-stranded ribonucleic acid (RNA) arbovirus, family *Flaviviridae*
  - Most commonly spread by mosquitos; birds are usually primary host
  - Typically bilateral multifocal chorioretinitis, occurring in almost 80% of patients with acute WNV infection associated with neurologic illness
  - Originally found in Uganda; US origins in New York 1999, now throughout North and South America
- Symptoms
  - Most have no ocular symptoms
  - Mild blurring
  - Floaters
- Laterality
  - Typically bilateral
- Course
  - Typically self-limiting but may have permanent sequelae

C. S. Foster et al. (eds.), *Uveitis*, https://doi.org/10.1007/978-3-030-52974-1_39

- Age of onset
  - Any
- Gender/race
  - Any/more prevalent in endemic areas
- Systemic associations
  - West Nile fever

Exam: Ocular

Anterior Segment

- Anterior uveitis associated with vitritis
- Nystagmus
- Strabismus

Posterior Segment

- Chorioretinal lesions in the midzone and/or periphery in almost all eyes
  - May be congenital
- Prominent linear clustering of chorioretinal lesions
  - Related to course of retinal nerve fibers, suggesting a contiguous spread of CNS disease
- Retinal hemorrhages
- Focal or diffuse occlusive vasculitis
- Optic neuritis

Exam: Systemic

- Flu-like syndrome
- Neurologic involvement
  - Meningitis, encephalitis
  - Poliomyelitis-like disease
  - Cranial nerve palsies
- Also hepatitis, pancreatitis, myocarditis, cardiac dysrhythmia, nephritis

Imaging

- OCT – hyperreflective lesions from ONL to RPE with focal disruption; atrophic changes
- FAF – hypofluorescent or hyper autofluorescent lesions comparable to exam
- FA – early hypofluorescence and late staining of the chorioretinal lesions; inactive lesions appear with a typical "target like appearance" on FA with central hypofluorescence and peripheral hyperfluorescence
- ICG shows multiple well-delineated hypocyanescent lesions

Laboratory and Radiographic Testing

- Serology – WNV-specific IgG, IgM (most common)
  - Cross-reactions of flaviviruses common
- WNV PCR
- CSF – WNV IgM, pleocytosis
  - Essential with suspected neurologic involvement
- CBC with differential
  - Leukocytosis, lymphocytopenia, thrombocytopenia, anemia
- Plaque reduction neutralization test
- Magnetic resonance imaging (MRI) to detect neurologic involvement

Differential Diagnosis

- Syphilis
- Tuberculosis
- Sarcoidosis
- Idiopathic multifocal choroiditis
- Histoplasmosis
- Birdshot retinochoroiditis

Treatment

- No definitive treatment

Referral/Co-management

- Infectious Disease
- Neurology
- Report to CDC

Dengue Fever (DFV)

Overview

- Definition
  - Single-stranded RNA arbovirus, five types, family *Flaviviridae*
    - Subsequent infection with a different type may increase risk of severe complications
  - Commonly spread by mosquitos in tropical climates
  - Typically macular or foveal retinitis +/– hemorrhage which may occur in up to 10% of patients

- Symptoms
  - Blurring
  - Scotomas
  - Floaters
  - Less commonly redness, pain
- Laterality
  - Bilateral asymmetric
- Course
  - Acute onset of symptoms
  - Self-limiting with permanent sequelae
- Age of onset
  - Any
- Gender/race
  - Any/more prevalent in endemic areas (tropical)
- Systemic associations
  - Dengue fever

Exam: Ocular

Anterior Segment

- Anterior uveitis
- Opsoclonus (with neurologic involvement)

Posterior Segment

- Yellow subretinal dots, RPE mottling, foveolitis
- Retinal hemorrhages, retinal vascular sheathing
  - CRAO or BRAO
- Vitritis
- Retinochoroiditis
- Less common
  - Choroidal effusion, choroidal neovascularization
  - Optic disc swelling, optic neuritis
  - May cause panophthalmitis (rare)

Exam: Systemic

- Asymptomatic
- Classic dengue fever (high fever, severe headache, myalgias, arthralgias, nausea, vomiting, maculopapular rash)
  - Less common
    - Dengue hemorrhagic fever – hemorrhage, low platelets
    - Dengue shock syndrome – severe hypotension
- Encephalopathy

Imaging

- OCT: focal outer neurosensory retina–RPE thickening corresponding to the round, foveal yellowish lesion seen clinically (foveolitis)
- FA: prominent retinal vascular leakage, blocked fluorescence due to retinal hemorrhages and retinal–venular occlusion
- ICG: hypofluorescent spots corresponding to the subretinal lesions; large choroidal vasculopathy with hypercyanescence and leakage also common

Laboratory and Radiographic Testing

- IgM antibody capture ELISA
- Dengue group-specific NS1 monoclonal antibody (ELISA)
- CBC with differential

Differential Diagnosis

- Sarcoidosis
- Diabetic retinopathy
- Acute retinal pigment epitheliitis
- Syphilis
- Tuberculosis

Treatment

- No specific therapy
- Supportive therapy for uveitis, corticosteroid
- Vaccination recommended for those previously infected
- Systemic involvement may require hospitalization, transfusion
- Avoid NSAIDs due to risk of hemorrhage

Referral/Co-management

- Infectious disease
- Neurology with suspected encephalopathy
- Report to CDC

Chikungunya (CHK)

Overview

- Definition
  - Single-stranded RNA arbovirus, family *Togaviridae*
  - Commonly spread by mosquitos in tropical climates
  - Can be both endemic and epidemic, has occurred in Western nations
    Risk of death 1:1000
  - Systemic viral infection that may lead to a variety of ocular manifestations, most commonly uveitis
- Symptoms
  - Blurring
  - Redness
  - Light sensitivity
  - Pain
  - Floaters
  - Diplopia
- Laterality
  - Bilateral more than unilateral
- Course
  - Ocular involvement in acute disease
  - Less commonly initially manifest during chronic infection
- Age of onset
  - Any
- Gender/race
  - Any/more prevalent in endemic areas (tropical)
- Systemic associations
  - Chikungunya fever

Exam: Ocular

Anterior Segment
- Acute anterior uveitis (mimic herpetic anterior uveitis) – most common
  - May have hypopyon
  - Elevated IOP
- Keratitis, stromal edema
- Episcleritis, scleritis
- Conjunctivitis
- Cranial nerve palsies

Posterior Segment
- Mild vitritis
- Multifocal retinitis, retinal and macular edema, retinal hemorrhages

- Neuroretinitis
- Optic neuritis
- Central retinal artery occlusion
- Exudative retinal detachment
- Panophthalmitis

Exam: Systemic

- Findings associated with Chikungunya fever
  - Acute fever, severe arthralgia, skin rash
  - May have myocarditis, hepatitis, neurologic involvement

Imaging

- OCT: areas of hyper-reflectivity with after-shadowing; CME; retinal detachment; atrophic changes
- FA: early hypofluorescence with late-phase widespread retinal vascular leakage, staining of retinal infiltrates, and optic disc hyperfluorescence; capillary non-perfusion
- VF: arcuate or central scotomas, may be multifocal, cross-midline

Laboratory and Radiographic Testing

- Real-time PCR
- IgM serology

Differential Diagnosis

- Herpetic keratouveitis
- ANCA vasculitis
- Sarcoidosis
- Syphilis
- Tuberculosis

Treatment

- No definitive treatment for systemic disease
- Topical corticosteroids and cycloplegia for anterior segment manifestations
- Systemic corticosteroid therapy for more severe cases, that is, panuveitis, optic neuritis

Referral/Co-management

- Infectious Disease
- Others depending on systemic involvement
- Report to CDC

Zika Virus (ZKV)

Overview

- *Definition:*
  - Single-stranded RNA arbovirus, family *Flaviviridae*
  - Transmitted via mosquitos, sexual contact, pregnancy, transfusion
    Contagious 1–2 weeks after infection (also shed in tears)
  - First seen in Zika Forest, Uganda, 1947; spread to the Americas around 2007
- *Symptoms:*
  - Blurring, mild to severe
- *Laterality*
  - Unilateral or bilateral
- *Course*
  - Sub-acute, self-limiting
- *Age of onset*
  - Any; may also be congenital
- *Gender/race*
  - Any/more prevalent in endemic areas
- *Systemic association:*
  - Zika fever

Exam: Ocular

Anterior Segment

- None typical

Posterior Segment

- Grey perifoveal bull's-eye maculopathy
- Congenital
  - Retinal hemorrhages
  - Optic disc hypoplasia
  - Chorioretinal scarring, "torpedo maculopathy"
  - Vascular attenuation

Exam: Systemic

- May be asymptomatic
- Mild fever, rash, joint pain
- Guillain-Barré syndrome (rare)
- Congenital ZKV with microcephaly, brain malformations

Imaging (Only the Relevant Ones)

- OCT: disruptions in outer retina, RPE which may resolve
- FA: early hypofluorescence, late hyperfluorescence of macular lesion

Laboratory and Radiographic Testing

- PCR of serum, urine, saliva, tears, CSF while acutely ill
  - May be unable to perform if symptoms more than 7 days
- Serologic testing for ZKV IgM if symptoms >7 days
- Plaque reduction neutralization test (PRNT)
  - Subject to cross-reactivity with flaviviruses

Differential Diagnosis

- Acute idiopathic maculopathy

Treatment

- No definitive treatment
- Vaccines are currently in clinical trials
- Avoid sexual contact for 6 months post infection

Referral/Co-management

- Infectious Disease
- Report to CDC

Presumed Ocular Histoplasmosis Syndrome

40

Overview

- Definition
  - Ocular syndrome of peripheral punched out chorioretinal lesions (histo spots), peripapillary atrophy, macular scarring with or without choroidal neovascular membranes and absence of vitritis
  - Presumed exposure to the dimorphic fungus *Histoplasma capsulatum*
    - Grows in soil (mold) and inside animals/birds (yeast)
    - Endemic in valleys of Ohio and Mississippi Rivers, the "Histo belt"
- Symptoms
  - Asymptomatic mostly
  - Scotomas
  - Blurring
  - Metamorphopsia
  - Rarely photopsias
- Laterality
  - Typically unilateral, bilateral in up to 12%
- Course
  - Chronic, indolent
  - Acute symptomatic onset of secondary complications, choroidal neovascular membrane (CNV)
- Age of onset
  - Median age 36, may be present much earlier undetected
- Gender/race
  - No gender or racial predilection of overall disease
    - Disciform macular type more common in Caucasians
    - Bilateral more common in men
- Systemic association
  - Not in association with disseminated systemic histoplasmosis

C. S. Foster et al. (eds.), *Uveitis*, https://doi.org/10.1007/978-3-030-52974-1_40

Exam: Ocular

Anterior Segment

- No associated findings

Posterior Segment

- Clear vitreous
- Disseminated choroiditis, "histo spots," 4–8 per eye
  - Typical (inactive)
    - Small, circular depigmented and atrophic chorioretinal scars
      - 0.2–0.7DD, "punched-out" lesions
    - Mid-periphery and posterior to the equator
    - +/− central pigmented clump
  - Atypical (active)
    - Creamy yellow lesions, slightly elevated, in mid-periphery
    - More prone to develop CNV
  - Linear streaks (5% of patients)
    - Typical spots near equator that run in linear patterns parallel to the ora serrata
- Maculopathy, disciform macular scar
  - Old raised fibrovascular scar in macula, often a result of CNV
    - Or can be similar to histo spots
  - Active lesions at the edge of old lesions
- Peripapillary chorioretinal degeneration
  - Pigmented changes typical
  - +/− CNV in 11%
- Less common
  - Subretinal hemorrhage
  - Vitreous hemorrhage
  - "Disappearing lesions"
    - Histo spots may spontaneously resolve

Exam: Systemic

- None

Imaging (Only the Relevant Ones)

- OCT: disruption of external limiting membrane (ELM), ellipsoid and retinal pigment epithelium (RPE)/Bruch's membrane; pigment epithelial detachment (PED); CNV
- FAF: may detect small, nonpigmented macular chorioretinal scars

- FA: Classic CNV findings; window defects; active lesions show late hyperfluorescence
- ICG: increased hypercyanescence in affected choriocapillaris

Laboratory and Radiographic Testing

- Clinical diagnosis based on exam findings
- Chest X-ray, CT
- Serologic testing
  - Ancillary testing performed historically
    - Histoplasmin skin test
    - Histoplasma complement fixation test
  - HLA-B7 association

Differential Diagnosis

- White dot syndromes
  - Multifocal choroiditis and panuveitis (MCP)
  - Punctate inner choroidopathy (PIC)
  - Acute posterior multifocal placoid pigment epitheliopathy (APMPPE)
  - Multiple evanescent white dot syndrome (MEWDS)
- Idiopathic choroidal neovascularization
- Age-related macular degeneration
- Choroidal rupture
- Angioid streaks
- Central serous retinopathy
- Myopic degeneration
- Peripapillary coloboma
- Sarcoidosis
- Toxoplasmosis

Treatment

- Corticosteroids for active lesions
  - Systemic or periocular
- Intraocular anti-vascular endothelial growth factor (VEGF) agents or photodynamic therapy (PDT) for subfoveal and juxtafoveal CNV
- Laser photocoagulation for extrafoveal CNV
- Subretinal surgery not routinely performed for submacular CNV
  - High recurrence afterward

Referral/Co-management

- None typical

Candidiasis

41

Overview

- Definition
  - Intraocular candida infection, mainly endogenous, that might produce choroiditis, retinitis, or endophthalmitis

    Candida chorioretinitis: the presence of focal, deep, white infiltrative chorioretinal lesions with no evidence of vitreous involvement, except for vitreous haze

    Candida endophthalmitis: chorioretinitis with extension to the vitreous or a vitreous abscess manifesting as an intravitreal ball
- Symptoms
  - May be asymptomatic with peripheral lesions
  - Mild ocular discomfort
  - Red eye
  - Floaters
  - Slowly progressing visual loss
- Laterality
  - More frequently bilateral
- Course
  - Indolent and progressive
- Age of onset
  - No specific age group affected
- Gender/race
  - No gender or racial predilection
- Systemic association
  - Diabetes mellitus
  - Renal failure on dialysis
  - Endocarditis
  - HIV/AIDS

C. S. Foster et al. (eds.), *Uveitis*, https://doi.org/10.1007/978-3-030-52974-1_41

  - Malignancy
  - Systemic immunosuppression for autoimmune disorders or organ transplantation
  - Chronic corticosteroids use
  - Recent hospitalization and surgery
  - Indwelling catheter
  - Intravenous drug abuse

Exam: Ocular

Anterior Segment

- Conjunctival injection
- Anterior chamber cells and hypopyon

Posterior Segment

- Multifocal white, infiltrative, well-circumscribed lesions less than 1 mm in diameter, distributed throughout the post-equatorial fundus and associated with overlying vitreous cellular inflammation
- Vitreous cells and exudates
- Intraretinal hemorrhages
- Vascular sheathing
- Papillitis

Exam: Systemic

- Ranges from asymptomatic to lethal
- Fever, fatigue, loss of appetite
- Mucocutaneous lesions
- Dysphagia
- Disseminated intravascular coagulation
- Septic shock leading to multi-organ failure

Imaging

- FA
  - Highlights characteristic chorioretinal lesions, vascular and optic nerve leakage

Laboratory and Radiographic Testing

- Blood, urine, indwelling catheter cultures
- Anterior chamber (AC) tap has low yield
- Pars Plana Vitrectomy (PPV) is more reliable in speciating organisms

Differential Diagnosis

- Toxoplasma retinochoroiditis
- Bacterial endogenous endophthalmitis
- Viral retinitis
- Pars planitis

Treatment

- Chorioretinitis without vitreous involvement may be managed with systemic anti-fungal therapy only; treatment duration varies, but at least 4–6 weeks
  - Amphotericin B (AMB)
    0.5–1.0 mg/kg/day
    Not preferred due to poor ocular penetration and toxicity, most notably nephrotoxicity
  - Fluconazole
    6–12 mg/kg loading dose, then 6–12 mg/kg daily
    Excellent ocular penetration and systemic safety
  - Voriconazole
    6 mg/kg for 2 doses, then 4 mg/kg BID
    Excellent ocular penetration and systemic safety
    May have better efficacy for *Candida* and *Aspergillus* than the other meds, but much more expensive
- Candida endophthalmitis should be treated with a combination of systemic and intravitreal anti-fungal agents, with or without vitrectomy
  - Amphotericin 5–10 μg/0.1 cc
  - Voriconazole 10 0 μg/0.1 cc

Referral/Co-management

- Infectious Disease

Coccidioidomycosis

42

Overview

- Definition
  - A fungal infection acquired via inhalation of spores of soil-dwelling fungi *Coccidioides immitis* (California) and *Coccidioides posadasii* (elsewhere), often after disruption of contaminated soils, that is, construction/excavation, dust storms, earthquakes
  - Also known as San Joaquin Valley fever, or simply Valley fever
  - Primary infection manifests most frequently as a community-acquired pneumonia (chest pain, cough, fever, with or without hemoptysis that suggests pulmonary cavity) but can cause systemic symptoms (drenching sweats, weight loss, fatigue) for weeks to months, skin lesions (erythema nodosum or erythema multiforme), and rheumatologic symptoms ("desert rheumatism"), or can be entirely asymptomatic
  - In high-risk individuals, infection can disseminate to the skin, bone, soft tissues, meninges, and sometimes the eye
- Symptoms
  - Pain
  - Redness
  - Photophobia
  - Floaters
  - Blurry vision
- Laterality
  - Bilateral
- Course
  - Progressive ocular inflammation unless systemic or intraocular antifungal is given in a timely fashion
  - Anterior segment involvement generally fares worse than posterior, with majority requiring enucleation owing to blindness and pain

C. S. Foster et al. (eds.), *Uveitis*, https://doi.org/10.1007/978-3-030-52974-1_42

- Age of onset
  - Middle-aged and elderly
- Gender/race
  - No gender predilection
  - Common in semi-arid areas, where disease is endemic, including Southwest United States (California and Arizona), Northern Mexico, and Central/South America
    - Travel history is crucial in diagnosis
- Systemic association
  - Asymptomatic (60%)
  - Acute, self-limited pulmonary illness (40%)
    - 1–3 weeks after inhalation of spores
    - Pleuritic chest pain, nonproductive cough, fever, malaise
    - Erythema nodosum affecting the lower extremities, as well as erythema multiforme in a necklace distribution: 3 days to 3 weeks after onset of symptoms
  - Chronic progressive pneumonia (5–10%)
    - Profound fatigue and night sweats lasting for several weeks to months
  - Disseminated disease (<1%)
    - Skin, bone, soft tissues, and meninges are common sites
    - May follow symptomatic or asymptomatic pulmonary infection
    - High-risk individuals: HIV/AIDS (70% mortality when +meningitis), immunosuppressed, diabetic, pregnant, neonates, elderly, and those of Filipino, Native American, Mexican, and African ancestry

Exam: Ocular

Typically localized to either anterior or posterior segment but rarely both

External

- Orbital inflammation
- Extraocular nerve palsies

Anterior Segment

- Blepharitis
- Keratoconjunctivitis
- Phlyctenular or granulomatous conjunctivitis
- Scleritis and episcleritis
- Zonal granulomatous iridocyclitis with iris nodules that often involve the angle structures

Posterior Segment

- Posterior uveitis with diffuse choroiditis
- Optic atrophy and juxtapapillary choroidal infiltrates with overlying retinal hemorrhage
- Vitritis
- Perivascular sheathing
- Small peripheral scars with central hypopigmentation (increased CNV risk)

Exam: Systemic

- Scattered rales with or without areas of dullness to percussion over lung fields
- Erythema nodosum
- Erythema multiforme
- Arthralgias

Imaging

- OCT
  - Juxtapapillary choroidal infiltrates and overlying retinal edema
  - Spherical opacities at Bruch's membrane in the macula with CME and hard exudates
- FA
  - Late staining of peripheral chorioretinal scars
  - Macular leakage
  - Potential CNV associated with scars
- ICG
  - Highlights juxtapapillary and other less apparent choroidal infiltrates

Laboratory and Radiographic Testing

- Nonspecific
  - Eosinophilia (>5%) in about 25% of patients; degree of eosinophilia can be high
  - Chest X-ray/CT for pneumonitis and hilar adenopathy, thin-walled cavities, nodules
- Specific
  - Skin test positive for 1 month after onset: coccidioidin or spherulin antigens
    - Induration >5 mm diameter after 36 hours is considered positive
    - As with PPD testing for tuberculosis (TB), this type of skin testing is not helpful for diagnosing current illness, as it remains positive after infection has cleared

  - Serology
    - EIA/immunodiffusion, with titer measurement
    - Complement-fixing serum IgG anti-coccidioidal antibodies form by 3 months post infection and may persist for 6–8 months, but serology may be negative in immunocompromised hosts
  - PCR testing for *Coccidioides immitis*
  - Biopsy of skin/ocular lesions, or anterior chamber/vitreous tap to identify organism
    - Spherule and endospores best seen on Grocott's methenamine silver (GMS) but also visible on periodic acid Schiff and H&E
  - Culture (sputum, skin, ocular, central nervous system [CNS], etc.): important to alert the clinical laboratory about clinical concern for *Coccidioides*, as laboratory exposure can transmit infection to staff
  - Antigen testing: can be positive in urine, blood, cerebrospinal fluid (CSF), most helpful in immunocompromised hosts who are sero-negative

Differential Diagnosis (Ocular Disease)

- Presumed ocular histoplasmosis syndrome
- Cryptococcosis
- Tuberculosis

Treatment

- Observation and supportive care
  - Immunocompetent individuals with mild respiratory illness or asymptomatic lung nodules
- PO fluconazole or itraconazole (duration: months)
  - Nonpregnant patients with severe or persistently symptomatic disease
  - Nonpregnant patients who are at high risk for dissemination (immunocompromised hosts, diabetics, elderly/frail, underlying cardiopulmonary conditions, etc.)
- Intravenous (IV) amphotericin B, sometimes in combination with azole
  - Pregnant patients who require treatment (azoles are contraindicated in first trimester but may be considered later in pregnancy)
  - Patients with rapidly progressive pulmonary disease
  - Patients with severe disseminated disease (bones/joints, meninges)
- Surgical debridement of infected lung cavities or bones/joints
- Endogenous endophthalmitis (+/− concurrent PPV)
  - Amphotericin 5–10 μg/0.1 cc
  - Voriconazole 100 μg/0.1 cc

Referral/Co-management

- Infectious Disease
- Pulmonology

Cryptococcosis

43

Overview

- Definition
  - Fungal infection caused by yeast *Cryptococcus* species, most commonly affecting the lungs and central nervous system (CNS)
    - *C. neoformans* is most common, predominantly affecting immunosuppressed patients
    - *C. gattii* is the second most common, predominantly affecting immunocompetent patients in tropical climates, but there have been clusters of cases in British Columbia, Canada, and in the American Pacific Northwest, as well as sporadic cases in other regions of the United States, Asia, Africa, Mexico, and South America
  - Ubiquitous in soil, decaying wood, and bird droppings; transmitted via inhalation of aerosolized fungus
  - Most common cause of fungal meningitis in immunocompromised hosts
  - Most common ocular fungal infection in HIV/AIDS patients
- Symptoms
  - Blurry vision
  - Floaters
  - Photophobia
  - Pain
  - Diplopia
- Laterality
  - Bilateral
- Course
  - Insidious onset with poor visual prognosis
  - Ocular disease often follows meningitis immediately via hematogenous dissemination or direct extension from leptomeninges

C. S. Foster et al. (eds.), *Uveitis*, https://doi.org/10.1007/978-3-030-52974-1_43

- Age of onset
  - Extremely rare in prepubescent patients
- Gender/race
  - More common in males, even before the AIDS epidemic
  - Worldwide distribution
- Systemic association
  - Pulmonary disease: may be asymptomatic, or presents like pneumonia with shortness of breath, cough, chest pain, and fever
  - Cryptococcal meningitis: intracranial hypertension, headaches, lethargy; altered mental status portends poor prognosis
  - Skin disease: typically reflects systemic infection/disseminated disease, but skin lesions may precede systemic symptoms by 2–8 months; range of skin lesions is broad, including molluscum contagiosum-like umbilicated papules; pustules; soft subcutaneous masses and ulcers
  - Hematogenous dissemination to the heart, liver, prostate, bone, and mucus membranes

Exam: Ocular

Anterior Segment

Occurs if posterior segment infection is not treated promptly

- Conjunctival granulomas and injection
- Keratitis
- Scleral abscess
- Inflammatory iris masses with cells and flare, keratic precipitates, posterior synechiae

Posterior Segment

- Focal or multifocal chorioretinitis with yellowish to white, elevated, subretinal lesions
- Significant vitritis with fluffy exudates
- Perivascular sheathing
- Subretinal lesions with localized serous retinal detachment

Neuro-ophthalmological

- Papilledema
- Ocular motor palsies (sixth nerve most common)
- Facial nerve palsy

- Nystagmus
- Ptosis

Exam: Systemic

- CNS: fever (though not always present), mental status change, headache, memory loss, personality change, neck rigidity, photophobia, cranial neve palsies; symptoms can be acute or subacute/chronic
- Skin: painless papules or pustules mostly on head and neck that become ulcerated; can have various appearances resembling acne, molluscum contagiosum, or even basal cell carcinoma
- Pulmonary: cough, tachypnea

Laboratory and Radiographic Testing

- Serum cryptococcal antigen
- Chest X-ray/computed tomography (CT)
- CNS imaging (CT or magnetic resonance imaging [MRI]) prior to LP if there is concern for increased intracranial pressure based on history/physical exam
- Lumbar puncture for measurement of opening pressure and cerebrospinal fluid (CSF) analysis; CSF often shows lymphocytosis but absolute numbers of white blood cells (WBCs) are often lower than for other types of meningitis (e.g., <50 cells/microliter), elevated protein, decreased glucose; Immunocompromised patients may have a normal CSF profile. Encapsulated yeasts can be seen on India ink smears in patients with high organism burden. CSF cryptococcal antigen testing yields a titer that informs about the fungal burden and prognosis
- Fungal culture of CSF, sputum, blood, and urine
- Fixed-tissue staining with calcofluor white and Grocott methenamine silver (GMS)

Differential Diagnosis

- *Pneumocystis* choroiditis
- Coccidioidomycosis (Valley fever)
- Toxoplasma retinochoroiditis
- Viral retinitis (HSV, VZV, CMV)
- Candidiasis
- Endogenous bacterial endophthalmitis
- Syphilis
- Tuberculosis
- Sarcoidosis
- Intraocular lymphoma

Treatment (Dosing Is for Patients with Normal Renal Function)

- Immunocompetent patients
  - Mild–moderate pulmonary or other localized disease without disseminated infection
    PO fluconazole 400 mg/day for 6–12 months
  - More severe localized disease or meningitis
    Amphotericin B 0.7–1.0 mg/kg intravenous (IV) qd (or liposomal amphotericin B 3–4 mg/kg IV qd) and PO flucytosine 25 mg/kg q6h for several weeks, then
    PO fluconazole 400 mg/day
  - Meningitis/ocular disease
    Amphotericin B 0.7–1.0 mg/kg IV qd (or liposomal amphotericin B 3–4 mg/kg IV qd) and PO flucytosine 25 mg/kg q6h for 2–4 weeks, then
    PO fluconazole 400 mg/day for 8 weeks, then
    PO fluconazole 200 mg/day for at least 6–12 months
- Patients with AIDS: all require treatment
  - Mild-to-moderate pulmonary disease
    PO fluconazole 400 mg/day for 6–12 months
  - Meningitis/severe pulmonary disease/intraocular infection
    Amphotericin B 0.7–1.0 mg/kg IV qd (or liposomal amphotericin B 3–4 mg/kg IV qd) and PO flucytosine 25 mg/kg q6h >2 weeks, then
    PO fluconazole 400 mg/day for 10 weeks, then
    Long-term maintenance therapy with PO fluconazole 200 mg/day for at least 1 year and until CD4 >100, with undetectable viral load on antiviral therapy for at least 3 months but must continue to monitor and restart if CD4 count falls to <100 cells/microliter and/or the serum cryptococcal antigen titers rise
- For severe ocular disease, PPV with intravitreal voriconazole 100 μg/0.1 ml should be performed

Referral/Co-management

- Infectious Disease
- Neurology/neurosurgery for patients with increased intracranial pressure, which is typically a very challenging problem that requires frequent LPs or lumbar/ventricular drains

Sporotrichosis

44

Overview

- Definition
  - Rare infectious caused by dimorphic fungus *Sporothrix schenkii*
  - Also known as rose gardener's disease
  - Typically spread via traumatic contact with flora, especially rose thorns
  - Other sources include sphagnum moss, hay bales, animals (cats), fish, insects
  - May be inhaled (uncommon)
  - Most ocular cases are exogenous, but some may be endogenous
- Symptoms
  - Swelling involving skin around eye
  - Redness
  - Pain
  - Photophobia
  - Visual decline
- Laterality
  - Typically unilateral
- Course
  - Acute, severe if untreated
- Age of onset
  - Typically adult
  - Pediatric or adolescent involvement in endemic/tropical areas
- Gender/race
  - Any/no racial predilection but more common in endemic areas
- Systemic association
  - Lymphocutaneous infection at site of inoculation
  - Systemic findings may present

C. S. Foster et al. (eds.), *Uveitis*, https://doi.org/10.1007/978-3-030-52974-1_44

Exam: Ocular

Anterior Segment

- Nontender hard round nodules on skin, eyelids – most common
- Conjunctival granulomas
- Anterior uveitis, hypopyon
- Iris nodules
- Posterior synechiae
- Cataract
- Corneal ulcer
- Scleritis
- Orbital cellulitis
- Phthisis

Posterior Segment

- Vitritis, fluffy vitreous opacities
- Retinal granuloma
- Endophthalmitis (endogenous)
- Glaucoma

Exam: Systemic

- Cutaneous nodular pink, nontender lesions usually along lymphatics
  - May become black or necrotic (sporotrichitic chancre)
- Mediastinal lymphadenopathy
- Disseminated disease in immunocompromised patients
  - Central nervous system (CNS) (meningitis), arthritis

Imaging (Only the Relevant Ones)

- Anterior segment photography: can document the lesion and progression/ response to treatment
- Ultrasound- evaluated the status of posterior segment in media haze (in diseases including endophthalmitis)
- FFA and OCT: evaluates involvment of the posterior segment when reasonable media clarity is present

Laboratory and Radiographic Testing

- Culture from cutaneous or conjunctival lesion on Sabouraud's agar
  - Difficult to isolate from serum, urine, aqueous, vitreous
- Serology for *S. schenckii* IgM, IgG
- Intradermal skin testing no longer used

Differential Diagnosis

- Bartonella
- Tuberculosis
- Syphilis
- Other fungal infections (coccidiomycosis, histoplasmosis, candidiasis)
- Sarcoidosis
- Herpes simplex
- Atypical mycobacteria – leprosy
- Tularemia
- Nocardia
- Parasitic– leishmaniasis

Treatment

- Topical amphotericin for cutaneous lesions
- Intravitreal voriconazole, amphotericin for intraocular involvement
  - Pars plana vitrectomy to reduce fungal burden
- Disseminated disease – PO itraconazole (200 mg daily to BID) for 3–6 months
  - 2–4 weeks after all lesions resolved
  - Also fluconazole, voriconazole, amphotericin
- Local heat application
- Supersaturated solution of potassium iodide (oral)
  - 5 drops TID increasing to 40–50 drops TID per tolerance

Referral/Co-management

- Infectious Disease
- Dermatology
- Pulmonology

Pneumocystosis

45

Overview

- Definition
  - Opportunistic infection of yeast-like fungus *Pneumocystis jirovecii* (previously *P. carinii*), mainly occurring in immunocompromised humans
  - Less common with widespread use of highly active antiretroviral therapy (HAART) and prophylaxis
  - Mainly causes choroidopathy, denotes poor systemic prognosis
  - Spread via inhalation of infectious organisms
- Symptoms
  - May be asymptomatic, even with foveal involvement
  - Mild blurring
- Laterality
  - 75% bilateral
- Course
  - Often diagnosed during routine exam or screening
  - Lesions may resolve without visual sequelae after treatment
- Age of onset
  - Typically adults
- Gender/race
  - No predilection
- Systemic association
  - Immunocompromised state, that is, HIV+ patients with CD4 count <50/mm

C. S. Foster et al. (eds.), *Uveitis*, https://doi.org/10.1007/978-3-030-52974-1_45

Exam: Ocular

Anterior Segment

- None, typically

Posterior Segment

- Multiple elevated, yellow-white, plaque-like deep lesions under vessels
  - Polylobar, may become confluent
  - Vessels not disturbed by lesions
  - Mostly in posterior pole, never anterior to equator
- No vitritis
- Serous retinal detachment

Exam: Systemic

- Signs of significant immunocompromised state
- Pneumonia

Imaging

- FA: hypofluorescence early and late homogenous staining of lesions with unclear borders
- Visual Field: depression corresponding to area of lesion

Laboratory and Radiographic Testing

- Elevated LFTs
- Decreased arteriolar blood gas
- Chest imaging shows pulmonary lesions (chest x-ray, CT)
- Bronchoalveolar lavage may allow detection of parasite with Giemsa, Gomori methenamine silver, or indirect immunofluorescence

Differential Diagnosis

- Tuberculosis
- Toxoplasmosis
- Candidiasis
- Cryptococcosis

- Mycobacterium avium intracellular
- Lymphoma
- Histoplasmosis
- Sarcoidosis
- Vogt-Koyanagi-Harada disease
- Sympathetic ophthalmia
- Progressive outer retinal necrosis

Treatment

- Induction therapy
  - TMX 15 mg/kg/day with SMX 75 mg/kg/day

  or
  - Pentamidine 4 mg/kg/day
- Prophylaxis – TMP-SMX with low CD4 count,
  - Aerosolized pentamidine as adjunct

Referral/Co-management

- Infectious Disease
- Pulmonology

Toxoplasmosis

46

Overview

- Definition
  - A protozoal disease caused by *Toxoplasma gondii*, contracted from cat feces, consumption of unfiltered water, or undercooked meat (especially pork, lamb, and venison). Infection can also be acquired via vertical transmission (from mother to fetus) and via receipt of an organ transplanted from an infected donor
  - Up to a third of the world's population is infected, but only a very small percentage manifest symptomatically
  - Ocular toxoplasmosis is the number one cause of infectious posterior uveitis in the world (>80% in some regions)
  - While chorioretinitis is common in all hosts, systemic disease is exceedingly rare in immunocompetent hosts
- Symptoms
  - Blurry vision
  - Floaters
  - Pain (from anterior uveitis and/or scleral involvement of retinochoroiditis)
  - Redness
  - Photophobia
  - Photopsia
- Laterality
  - Unilateral or bilateral (but simultaneous bilateral inflammation is extremely rare)

C. S. Foster et al. (eds.), *Uveitis*, https://doi.org/10.1007/978-3-030-52974-1_46

- Course
  - Retinochoroiditis is self-limited over 2–4 weeks in immunocompetent hosts but can recur in two-thirds of patients
  - Visual prognosis is favorable unless lesion affects macula or optic nerve; surprisingly, congenital macular scar may be associated with relatively good vision
  - Much more aggressive in immunocompromised hosts
- Age of onset
  - All ages affected, but more severe in older patients
  - Seroconversion increases with age: 5–30% of 10–19 years old are seropositive for *T. gondii*, and this goes up to 70% in those older than 50
- Gender/race
  - No gender or racial predilection
  - Higher prevalence in tropical areas close to sea level
- Systemic association
  - Congenital toxoplasmosis
    - Incidence of primary infection during pregnancy is <1%; among these, transplacental transmission risk increases with gestational age at the time of maternal infection, up to ~70% at 36 weeks
      - More severe clinical sequelae for the fetus when contracted early on in pregnancy (may lead to spontaneous abortion)
    - No risk of congenital infection from reactivation of latent toxoplasmosis during pregnancy in immunocompetent hosts; very small to no risk in immunocompromised hosts
    - Retinochoroiditis is the most common manifestation: often bilateral with macular involvement (15–40%)
    - Cerebrospinal fluid pleocytosis and elevated proteins (20%)
    - Intracranial calcifications (10%)
    - Anemia, thrombocytopenia, and jaundice at birth
    - Mental retardation, seizures, spasticity, sensorineural hearing loss are some severe neurologic sequelae
  - Acquired toxoplasmosis
    - Immunocompetent patients: only 10–20% ever develop symptoms, which are usually mild and nonspecific, and self-limited over 2–4 weeks
      - Lymphadenopathy, with mono-like illness: headache, malaise, sore throat, fatigue, fever, and night sweats
      - More severe (but unusual) symptoms: meningismus, meningoencephalitis, myalgias, arthralgias, abdominal pain, and maculopapular rash sparing palms and soles
      - Potentially lethal (but very rare) complications: encephalopathy, pneumonitis, myocarditis, polymyositis, hepatitis, and splenomegaly
    - Immunocompromised patients: many develop rapidly fatal disease if untreated
      - CNS disease (50%): encephalopathy, meningoencephalitis, and mass lesions

- Myocarditis
- Pneumonitis
- Disseminated disease with septic shock

Exam: Ocular

Anterior Segment

- Mild to severe granulomatous or non-granulomatous uveitis
- Elevated IOP (10–15%)

Posterior Segment

- Classic appearance ("headlight in the fog"): fluffy, focal necrotizing retinitis or retinochoroiditis adjacent to a variably pigmented chorioretinal scar, with significant overlying vitritis
  - Lesion size ranges from 1/10 disc diameters to large enough to span two quadrants of the fundus
  - Recurrent lesions are typically single and contiguous with old inactive scars, but can also recur at sites distant from the primary lesion or in the fellow eye
  - Vascular occlusion can occur if lesion involves vessels
  - Healed lesions are characterized by peripheral hyperpigmentation and central atrophy exposing the choroid and sclera; tractional bands may form between one scar to a neighboring scar or the optic disc; may be complicated by proliferative vitreoretinopathy and choroidal neovascularization
- Vascular sheathing typically involving veins but sometimes arteries (Kyrieleis arteriolitis)
- Optic atrophy
- Tractional or exudative retinal detachment

Atypical Forms

- Anterior uveitis without evidence of retinochoroiditis
- Punctate outer retinal toxoplasmosis
- Neuroretinitis
- Isolated optic neuritis
- Multifocal retinochoroiditis simulating acute retinal necrosis (ARN) (immunocompromised or recently acquired)
- Panophthalmitis (immunocompromised)

Exam: Systemic

- Enlarged lymph nodes (cervical [symmetrical, nontender] > suboccipital > supraclavicular > axillary > inguinal > mediastinal)
- Abdominal tenderness, hepatosplenomegaly
- Maculopapular rash (sparing palms and soles)
- Altered mental status, cerebellar signs, cranial nerve palsies, sensory abnormalities, weakness

Imaging

- OCT
  - Active lesion: hyperreflective retinal layers with posterior optical shadowing and overlying posterior hyaloid thickening
  - Healed lesion: atrophic retina with hyperreflectivity of the underlying choroid
- FA
  - Active lesion: early central hypofluorescence followed by late leakage from the margins; adjacent retinal vascular leakage
  - Healed lesion: variable early fluorescence depending on RPE proliferation or atrophy; late staining of margins
- ICG
  - Active lesion: early hyperfluorescence or hypofluorescence with late hyperfluorescence
  - Healed lesion: early and late hypofluorescence

Laboratory and Radiographic Testing

- Serum or ocular fluid anti–*T. gondii* IgG and IgM titers
  - In acute infection, IgM should be positive within a week of developing symptoms and persist for several weeks
  - IgG develops over the next 2–3 weeks and typically persists for life
  - Patients with positive IgM and negative IgG may have acute infection but may also have false-positive IgM results due to cross-reactivity with rheumatoid factor, antinuclear antibodies, or nonspecific binding in vitro. These patients should have repeat serologies checked 2–3 weeks later to assess for development of IgG, which confirms true acute infection
  - Patients with symptoms for more than 2 weeks who lack both toxoplasma IgG and IgM likely do not have toxoplasmosis
  - In reactivation disease, serum IgM antibodies are typically absent, while IgG antibodies are present
  - Goldmann-Witmer coefficient

$$C = \frac{\text{Antibody titer in aqueous humor}}{\text{Antibody titer in serum}} \times \frac{\text{Globulin titer in serum}}{\text{Globulin titer in aqueous humor}}$$

0.5–2: No anti-toxoplasma intraocular antibody (Ab) production
2–4: Possible intraocular Ab production
>4: Definitive intraocular Ab production

- Serum and ocular fluid *T. gondii* DNA PCR
  - Done in suspicious cases with negative serologic testing
- MRI or CT of brain
- Histopathology: tachyzoites or cysts may be seen in lymph nodes, brain tissue, or other infected organs

Differential Diagnosis

- Congenital disease: TORCH infections
- Endogenous fungal endophthalmitis
  - Candidiasis
  - Aspergillosis
  - Blastomycosis
- Subretinal abscess from endogenous bacterial endophthalmitis
- Viral retinitis
- Syphilis
- Tuberculosis
- Toxocariasis
- Sarcoidosis
- Lymphocytic choriomeningitis virus (LCMV)

Treatment

Treat at least 4–6 weeks, then reevaluate; consult Infectious Disease for pediatric dosing

- "Classic" therapy (nonpregnant adults)
  - Pyrimethamine: 100 mg on day 1, then 25–50 mg daily

    Access to pyrimethamine in the United States is currently difficult— it must be obtained through a program administered by the manufacturer or from a compounding pharmacy (www.daraprimdirect.com/how-to-prescribe). If this cannot be done promptly, then trimethoprim–sulfamethoxazole should be used until pyrimethamine is obtained
  - Sulfadiazine: 2 g loading dose on day 1, then 500 mg–1 g QID
  - Folinic acid (leucovorin): 5–25 mg/d based on neutrophil count
  - Congenital toxoplasmosis in newborn is treated 6–24 months

- Prophylaxis in HIV
  Pyrimethamine 25–75 mg daily
  Sulfadiazine 0.5–1 g QID
  Folinic acid 5–25 mg daily
- Trimethoprim/sulfamethoxazole
  - 160/800 mg BID, then every other day for 1 year
  - May be less effective than classic therapy, but a good alternative when retinochoroiditis is not threatening posterior pole or optic nerve
  - Can be used in late second or third trimester for maternal and fetal infections
- Atovaquone, preferably with pyrimethamine but alone if unable to give pyrimethamine
  - 1500 mg BID
  - Give with food to increase bioavailability
  - Excellent choice when patient has sulfa allergy
  - May need to treat for at least 3 months if giving without pyrimethamine
- Clindamycin
  - 300 mg q6–8 h
  - Intravitreal 1 mg/0.1 ml can be used in conjunction with systemic therapy when vision is threatened
- Azithromycin
  - 0.5–1 g daily
- Spiramycin
  - 1 g TID
  - Drug of choice during early pregnancy (<18 weeks gestation) due to concerns about teratogenicity with pyrimethamine–sulfadiazine in early pregnancy
  - Significantly lowers vertical transmission rate
  - Licensed in Canada and Europe but available in the United States only via the Food and Drug Administration (FDA) using an IND
- Prednisone
  - Indicated if active chorioretinitis threatens posterior pole or optic nerve, or if there is visually significant vitritis
  - Start 24–72 hours after antiparasitic therapy

Referral/Co-management

- Infectious Disease
- Ob-Gyn
- Neurology
- Cardiology
- Pulmonology

Acanthamoeba

47

Overview

- Definition
  - Ocular infection caused by the free-living amoeba *Acanthamoeba*, which is ubiquitous in water and soil
  - Typically affects the cornea, but can also involve the sclera, uvea, and other ocular tissues
  - Risk factors: contact lens wear with poor hygiene and homemade saline solution, corneal trauma, and exposure to contaminated water
- Symptoms
  - Severe pain and tearing far out of proportion of clinical signs
    Some cases have no pain
  - Decreased vision
- Laterality
  - Unilateral
- Course
  - Acute and progressive; poor visual prognosis if not treated early and aggressively
- Age of onset
  - All age groups affected
- Gender/Race
  - No gender predilection
  - Higher incidence in developing tropical countries
- Systemic association
  - In immunocompromised individuals, *Acanthamoeba* can enter the body via nasal passage or open wounds, and spread hematogenously to the central nervous system (CNS), causing fatal granulomatous amoebic encephalitis (GAE)

C. S. Foster et al. (eds.), *Uveitis*, https://doi.org/10.1007/978-3-030-52974-1_47

Exam: Ocular

Anterior Segment

- Acanthamoeba keratitis
  - Pseudodendritic epitheliopathy
  - Radial keratoneuritis
  - Ring infiltrates
  - Absence of purulent discharge (in contrast with bacterial keratitis)
- Granulomatous AC reaction with hypopyon in late stages
- Nodular scleritis if diagnosis is delayed by 2+ months
- Cataract and glaucoma are common complications

Posterior Segment

- Chorioretinitis is extremely rare

Exam: Systemic

- None

Imaging

- In vivo confocal microscopy to look for trophozoites and cysts

Laboratory and Radiographic Testing

- Cornea can be biopsied and processed to facilitate diagnosis:
  - Histopathology and staining with Giemsa, periodic acid–Schiff, methylene blue, or calcofluor white
  - Cultured on blood, chocolate, and non-nutrient agar with *E. coli* overlay
  - PCR for acanthamebal RNA (most sensitive)

Differential Diagnosis

- Bacterial, fungal, herpetic or sterile contact lens–associated keratitis
- Topical anesthetic abuse

Treatment

- Prevention is key: good contact lens fitting, frequent lens disinfection, and proper storage
- Combination of a topical biguanide (0.02% chlorhexidine and 0.02% polyhexamethyl biguanide) and a topical diamidine (propamidine isethionate and hexamidine), both of which are cysticidal
- Topical corticosteroid may be used judiciously in treatment-refractory cases where inflammation is profound
  - Antiameba therapy should be continued for at least 6 weeks after cessation of steroids
- Oral NSAIDs for scleritis and limbal inflammation
- Surgical treatment
  - Keratoplasty and cryotherapy with freeze-thaw-refreeze of the peripheral host cornea
  - Collagen crosslinking with ultraviolet (UV) light and riboflavin may be an adjuvant for treatment of medically refractive acanthamoeba keratitis

Referral/Co-management

- None

48 Giardia Lamblia

Overview

- Definition
  - Motile, flagellated protozoan responsible for giardiasis
  - Endemic to all climates
  - Spread through fecal-oral route and consumption of contaminated water and food, especially untreated drinking water while camping
  - Increased prevalence with immune deficiency
  - Ocular findings likely secondary to hypersensitivity reaction
- Symptoms
  - Blurring
  - Pain
  - Redness
  - Light sensitivity
  - Floaters
- Laterality
  - Unilateral or bilateral
- Course
  - Incubation period: 7–21 days
  - Ocular disease occurs with active systemic symptoms
  - Frequently self-limited disease, but prolonged, indolent course possible
- Age of onset
  - All age groups affected
- Gender/race
  - No gender or racial predilection
- Systemic association
  - Giardiasis

C. S. Foster et al. (eds.), *Uveitis*, https://doi.org/10.1007/978-3-030-52974-1_48

Exam: Ocular

Anterior Segment

- Anterior uveitis

Posterior Segment

- Choroiditis
- Salt-and-pepper retinopathy
- Vitelliform macular lesions
- Retinal hemorrhages
- Retinal arteritis
- Neuroretinitis
- Vitreous hemorrhage

Exam: Systemic

- Gastrointestinal – diarrhea, abdominal cramps, flatulence, nausea, bloating, anorexia, malabsorption of fat, failure to thrive, irritable bowel, functional dyspepsia
- Extra-intestinal (1/3rd of cases) – fatigue, chills, reactive arthritis (rare), ocular disease

Imaging

- OCT: sub-RPE vitelliform lesions with surrounding subretinal fluid
- FA: arteriolar leakage
- ICG: hypocyanescent spots
- ERG: normal

Laboratory and Radiographic Testing

- Stool samples with cysts and/or trophozoites
  - Multiple samples required (three), organism excreted intermittently
- Motile organisms in jejunal aspirate
- Small bowel biopsy with visualized cysts and/or trophozoites

Differential Diagnosis

- Whipple's disease
- Sarcoidosis

- Reactive arthritis
- Irritable bowel disease (IBD)-associated anterior uveitis

Treatment

- Mepacrine hydrochloride 100 mg TID for 5–7 days
- Metronidazole 400 mg TID for 5 days
- Ocular findings treated with topical, periocular and/or systemic corticosteroid

Referral/Co-management

- Infectious Disease
- Gastrointestinal

Trypanosomiasis 49

Overview

- Definition
  - A vector-borne disease caused by protozoal parasites of genus *Trypanosoma*, with two very different varieties in humans
  - Human African trypanosomiasis (HAT), or "sleeping sickness"
    Caused by *T. brucei rhodesiense* and *T. brucei gambiense* transmitted by infected tsetse flies found only in Africa
    Found only in sub-Saharan Africa, as tsetse fly is only vector
  - American trypanosomiasis, or Chagas disease
    T. cruzi transmitted by bloodsucking triatomine bugs, but can spread via blood transfusion, organ transplant, placental transfer, and oral route
    Found mainly in rural Central and South America, but the United States has 200,000–300,000 cases due to different transmission modes
- Symptoms
  - HAT: blurry vision, light sensitivity
  - Chagas disease: Lid swelling, no vision change
- Laterality
  - Unilateral or bilateral
- Course
  - If untreated, HAT is often fatal within months, while Chagas disease becomes chronic and lifelong
  - Ocular changes are post-inflammatory and not progressive
- Age of onset
  - All age groups affected
- Gender/race
  - No gender or racial predilection

C. S. Foster et al. (eds.), *Uveitis*, https://doi.org/10.1007/978-3-030-52974-1_49

- Systemic association
  - HAT
    Stage 1 (hematolymphatic)
    - 1–3 weeks after insect bite
    - Fever, headaches
    - Myalgia, arthralgia
    - Rash and swelling of hands and periocular areas

    Stage 2 (meningoencephalitic)
    - Parasites invade central nervous system (CNS), causing characteristic insomnia and daytime drowsiness, personality changes, gait imbalance, and seizures
    - Fatal if untreated
  - Chagas disease
    Acute stage
    - Starts 1–2 weeks after insect bite
    - Fever and diffuse lymphadenopathy
    - Rare lethal events from myocarditis and meningoencephalitis

    Indeterminate stage
    - Asymptomatic
    - Majority of patients
    - May last 10–20 years or indefinitely

    Chronic stage
    - 20–30% of cases
    - Cardiomyopathy is the most serious complication
    - Megaesophagus and megacolon

Exam: Ocular

HAT

- Interstitial keratitis

Chagas Disease

- Romaña's sign: periorbital swelling from bug bite or direct inoculation of bug feces
- Post-inflammatory parafoveal RPE atrophy without visual sequelae

Exam: Systemic

HAT

- Skin chancre at site of insect bite
- Diffuse, enlarged lymph nodes
- Neurological/mental status assessment

Chagas Disease

- Swelling around insect bite
- Cardiac and pulmonary exams for congestive heart failure
- Inquire about difficulty with swallowing and bowel movement

Imaging

- n/a

Laboratory and Radiographic Testing

HAT

- *T. b. rhodesiense*
  - Seen easily on blood smear, or lymph node and chancre aspirate
  - Serologic testing not widely used as diagnosis easily made with above
- *T. b. gambiense*
  - Difficult to detect in blood
  - Requires (posterior cervical) lymph node aspirate
  - Serologic testing is useful for screening, but diagnosis is based on microscopic detection
- *T. cruzi*
  - Seen easily on blood smear in acute stage
  - Serologic testing may be necessary in chronic stage
- Lumbar puncture
  - Necessary in all HAT patients to determine CNS involvement

Differential Diagnosis

- n/a

Treatment

Contact the Centers for Disease Control and Prevention (CDC) or World Health Organization (WHO) for specific treatment protocols

- HAT
  - Suramin
  - Pentamidine
  - Melarsopro

  - Nifurtimox
  - Eflornithine
- Chagas disease
  - Benznidazole
  - Nifurtimox

Referral/Co-management

- Infectious Disease
- Neurology
- Cardiology
- Gastroenterology

Other Vector-Borne Parasitic Infections 50

Leishmaniasis

Overview

- Definition
  - Caused by protozoa (*Leishmania* species) which are transmitted by bites of infected sand flies (various species including *Phlebotomus*)
  - "Neglected tropical disease" mostly affecting poorest populations
    - Risk factors include malnutrition, weak immune system, poverty, poor housing, populations displacement, and deforestation
  - Presentation and management vary by species and affected population
  - Three forms of disease exist:
    - Cutaneous (most common) (CL)
    - Mucosal/mucocutaneous (Espundia) (ML)
    - Visceral (Kala-azar, black fever, most severe) (VL)
- Symptoms
  - CL, ML – blurring, pain, redness, light sensitivity
  - VL – blurring, pain, redness, light sensitivity, floaters
- Laterality
  - Typically unilateral
- Course
  - Subacute onset with chronic self-limiting course
    - May have permanent sequelae in more severe disease
  - ML is often seen after untreated or unrecognized CL
- Age of onset
  - All age groups affected
- Gender/race
  - Any person in endemic area

C. S. Foster et al. (eds.), *Uveitis*, https://doi.org/10.1007/978-3-030-52974-1_50

- Systemic association
  - CL – skin lesions mostly in exposed areas, may be diffuse
  - ML – mucosal erosions
  - VL – multisystem involvement, potentially fatal

Exam: Ocular

Anterior Segment

- CL – lid or periocular ulcers, madarosis, ectropion, trichiasis, exposure keratopathy
- ML – lid lesions similar to chalazia, basal cell carcinoma; dacryocystitis; interstitial keratitis
- VL – same as in CL, ML; also bilateral anterior uveitis, cataract, phthisis

Posterior Segment

- CL, ML – none
- VL – panuveitis, RD (retinal detachment) with PVR (proliferative vitreoretinopathy), retinal hemorrhage, glaucoma

Exam: Systemic

- CL – single/multiple papules, nodules, ulcers with raised margins and depressed center, may scab; regional lymphangitis
- ML – mucosal erosions, perforated nasal septum, oral/pharyngeal ulcers
- VL – hepatosplenomegaly, fever, anemia, pancytopenia, lymphadenopathy, hypergammaglobulinemia, hypoalbuminemia; post-VL dermal leishmaniasis with skin lesions involving face, trunk and genitals

Imaging

- Fundus photograph, fundus fluorescein angiography, and optical coherence tomography: may be needed to evaluate the involvement of the posterior segment

Laboratory and Radiographic Testing

- Biopsy of involved tissue demonstrating protozoa (amastigotes) with light microscopy (gold standard)
  - CL, ML – skin and mucosal lesions
  - VL – bone marrow, splenic aspirate with high yield (latter may have potentially lethal complications and is thus avoided)

- VL – culture (Novy-MacNeal-Nicolle medium), deoxyribonucleic acid (DNA) PCR, and serologies (rk39 rapid test, Leishmania IgM/IgG)

Differential Diagnosis

- CL – infections including bacterial, fungal, viral; sporotrichosis; dermatologic malignancies including basal cell carcinoma; inflammatory disease including plaque psoriasis
- ML – granulomatosis with polyangiitis (previously Wegener's), lethal midline granuloma, polymorphic reticulosis, lymphoma, nasopharyngeal carcinoma
- VL – systemic infections including military tuberculosis (TB), syphilis, brucellosis, endocarditis; malignancy including lymphoma, leukemia

Treatment

- Preventative
  - Clothing, insect repellent, avoidance of nocturnal activities
  - Early diagnosis and treatment of infected individuals who may act as reservoir
  - Control insect breeding
  - Improvement of living conditions, nutrition, immunocompromised conditions (HIV)
- Therapy
  - Pentavalent ammonium compounds
    Sodium stibogluconate 20 mg/kg intravenous (IV) for 20 days (CL) or 28 days (VL)
  - Liposomal amphotericin B (VL)
    Immunocompetent – 3 mg/kg/day IV on days 1–5, 14, and 21
    Immunocompromised – 4 mg/kg/day IV on days 1–5, 10, 17, 24, 31, and 38
  - Conventional amphotericin B deoxycholate 0.5–1 mg/kg/day, total dose 15–20 mg/kg or more
  - Miltefosine (>12 yo) 50 mg BID (30–44 kg) or TID (>45 kg) for 28 days
    Contraindicated in pregnancy, defer conception by 5 months
  - CL – ketoconazole 600 mg/day for 28 days; itraconazole 200 mg BID for 28 days; fluconazole 200–400 mg/day for 6 weeks
  - Pentamidine, allopurinol, topical paromomycin
  - Topical steroid and cycloplegia for anterior uveitis
  - Systemic corticosteroid may help posterior ocular findings

Referral/Co-management

- Dermatology
- Primary Care
- Infectious Disease

Malaria

Overview

- Definition
  - Caused by protozoa *Plasmodium* and transmitted by mosquito
  - Intraerythrocytic parasite
  - Ocular involvement in 20–30%, typically severe malaria
  - *Plasmodium vivax* (Pv) causes milder disease than *P. falciparum* (Pf) which can be lethal (cerebral malaria)
- Symptoms
  - Blurring
  - Conjunctival discoloration
    - Hemorrhage
    - Yellowing
  - Pain
  - Light sensitivity
  - Floaters
- Laterality
  - Unilateral or bilateral
- Course
  - Typically present only in severe malaria
- Age of onset
  - All age groups affected
- Gender/race
  - Any/*any* person in endemic area
- Systemic association
  - Systemic malarial infection
    - Severe flu-like symptoms
    - Encephalopathy
    - May lead to convulsion, coma, or death

Exam: Ocular

Anterior Segment

- Subconjunctival hemorrhage
- Conjunctival yellowing
- Anterior uveitis

Posterior Segment

- Retinal hemorrhage, preretinal or intraretinal
- Roth spots
- Vitreous hemorrhage
- Retinal edema

- Retinal ischemia
- Retinal vasculitis, periphlebitis (poor prognosis)
- Papilledema and optic neuritis (poor prognosis)

Exam: Systemic

- Fever with chills and rigor at definite intervals
- Headache
- Fatigue
- Muscle ache
- Nausea and vomiting
- Orthostatic hypotension
- Hepatosplenomegaly, anemia, thrombocytopenia
- Severe cases (Pf)
  - High fever (>40 °C)
  - Tachycardia
  - Delirium
  - Cerebral malaria with diffuse symmetrical encephalopathy
    Potentially fatal

Imaging

- OCT: may help to locate the location of hemorrhage
- FA: retinal vascular or optic disc leakage, occlusion; blocking defects from hemorrhage
- VF: scotomas

Laboratory and Radiographic Testing

- Peripheral blood smear showing protozoa (schizonts) within red blood cells (RBCs)
- Rapid diagnostic stick tests
  - *P. falciparum* histidine–rich protein 2 (PfHRP2)
  - Plasmodium lactate dehydrogenase (PLDH) for pan-malaria group

Differential Diagnosis

- Infectious – bacterial, fungal, viral, or protozoal
- Collagen vascular disease

Malignancy

- Heat stroke

Treatment

- Pf
  - Quinine-based therapy
    Quinine 1 g (600 mg base) PO, then 500 mg (300 mg base) PO 6–8 hours later, then 500 mg (300 mg base) PO at 24 hours and 48 hours after the initial dosewith
    Pyrimethamine-sulfadoxine, or doxycycline or clindamycin
  - Artemether-lumefantrine
  - Atovaquone-proguanil
  - Mefloquine
- Pv
  - Chloroquine with primaquine
  - Dihydroartemisinin-piperaquine with primaquine
- *P. malariae*
  - Chloroquine

Referral/Co-management

- Infectious Disease
- Primary Care/ICU

SHAPU (Seasonal Hyperacute Panuveitis)

Overview

- Definition
  - Seasonal severe unilateral inflammation occurring every 2 years in autumn
  - Suspected relation to tussock moth; exact cause is unknown
  - Previously called “seasonal endophthalmitis”
- Symptoms
  - Blurring
  - White or red eye
  - Floaters
  - Lack of pain

- Laterality
  - Unilateral
- Course
  - Hyperacute, rapid progression to blindness/phthisis
- Age of onset
  - Typically pediatric
- Gender/race
  - No gender predilection
  - Only reported in Nepal
- Systemic association
  - None

Exam: Ocular

Anterior Segment

- Severe anterior uveitis
  - May have hypopyon/fibrinoid reaction
  - Non-granulomatous or granulomatous
- White pupillary reflex
- Shallow anterior chamber
- Non-dilating pupil
- Hypotony (malignant hypotension) very typical
- Rapid progression to phthisis in weeks

Posterior Segment

- Severe vitritis

Exam: Systemic

- No findings

Imaging

- Ultrasonography: used to evaluate the vitreous, retina and choroid

Laboratory and Radiographic Testing

- Vitreous or aqueous tap showing Streptococcus pneumonia, Acinetobacter spp., varicella-zoster virus, and anellovirus (torque teno virus, torque teno midi, or torque teno mini virus) in some cases
- A yet-undiagnosed infectious organism or severe allergic response to moth antigen may be involved in the etiopathogenesis

Differential Diagnosis

- Endophthalmitis – endogenous, exogenous, traumatic
- Acute retinal necrosis
- Intraocular TB
- Syphilis
- Toxoplasmosis
- Sarcoidosis
- Behcet's disease

Treatment

- Early PPV (pars plana vitrectomy) only successful method of salvaging vision reported
  - Intraocular antibiotic, antiviral can be given after surgery
- Supportive care with topical antibiotic, steroid, cycloplegia

Referral/Co-management

- Microbiology
- Infectious Disease

51 Toxocariasis

Overview

- Definition
  - A zoonotic disease caused by ocular invasion of second-stage larvae of *Toxocara canis* or *Toxocara cati*, whose definitive hosts are dogs and cats, respectively
  - Contacts with dogs (especially puppies) and cats are risk factors, as these animals can carry embryonated eggs in their fur, but the most common route of infection is ingestion of soil/sand or fresh vegetables or fruits contaminated with embryonated eggs that were passed in dog/cat feces. Infection can be acquired also via ingestion of undercooked meat contaminated with encapsulated larvae from an infected non-canine animal that has ingested these eggs
  - Associated with uveitis, retinal granuloma, and endophthalmitis, among other ocular lesions
- Symptoms
  - Young children do not always complain (must look for signs such as leukocoria and strabismus)
  - Blurry vision
  - Redness
  - Pain
  - Photophobia
  - Diplopia
- Laterality
  - Typically unilateral
- Course
  - Visual prognosis depends on subtypes
    - Peripheral granuloma: typically preserved central vision
    - Posterior pole granuloma: poor vision

C. S. Foster et al. (eds.), *Uveitis*, https://doi.org/10.1007/978-3-030-52974-1_51

    Chronic endophthalmitis: variable based on location of granuloma and inflammatory complications
  - Potentially lethal if infection affects brain, heart, and lungs
- Age of onset
  - Median age in the United States is about 8 years, but range is broad (1–60)
- Gender/race
  - Slight male predominance
  - Most cases reported in Southeastern United States, France, Austria, India, Japan, Korea, China, and Brazil
- Systemic association
  - Eosinophilia in only 10% of patients
  - Most infections are asymptomatic
  - Visceral larva migrans (VLM) – most common in young children
    - Pneumonitis and hepatitis common
    - Cardiac and CNS involvements rare but potentially lethal

Exam: Ocular

Three subtypes: peripheral granuloma, posterior pole granuloma, and chronic endophthalmitis

Peripheral Granuloma

- Varying degree of AC and vitreous inflammation, but typically quiet by the time of diagnosis
- Dense, white mass in retinal periphery
- Traction leads to classic appearance of retinal folds contiguous with optic nerve
- Rarely complicated by tractional or rhegmatogenous RD

Posterior Pole Granuloma

- Varying degree of AC and vitreous inflammation
- Intraretinal or subretinal, grayish mass measuring 500–3000 μm
- Rare CNV as late complication

Chronic Endophthalmitis

- Intraocular granulomatous inflammation may be intense in a quiet-appearing eye
- Hypopyon
- Posterior synechiae
- May be complicated by cataract, glaucoma, cyclitic membrane, RD, and phthisis bulbi

Exam: Systemic

- VLM
  - Fever, anorexia
  - Wheezes and rales, dyspnea, chronic nonproductive cough
  - Hepatosplenomegaly
  - Pruritic rash
  - Mental status changes

Imaging

- OCT
  - Subretinal mass
- Ultrasound
  - Vitreous bands contiguous with highly reflective mass
  - Thickening of ciliary body

Laboratory and Radiographic Testing

- Serum *Toxocara* Ab (ELISA) but this test is not as sensitive for Ocular Larva Migrans (OLM) as for VLM. Diagnosis of OLM generally is made based on findings on ophthalmologic exam
- Intraocular fluid and vitreous sample (only if diagnosis is unclear or patient needs surgery for ocular complications)
  - *Toxocara* Ab

    Ratio of (level of specific IgG in aqueous humor/level of specific IgG in serum) to (total IgG in aqueous humor/total IgG in serum) greater than 3.0 is considered diagnostic
  - Eosinophils
  - Fragments of *Toxocara*
- Serum eosinophil count is not typically elevated in ocular toxocariasis

Differential Diagnosis

- Retinoblastoma
- Pars planitis
- Infectious endophthalmitis
- Toxoplasmosis
- Retinopathy of prematurity
- Persistent fetal vasculature
- Coats disease
- Familial exudative vitreoretinopathy

Treatment

- Prevention
  - Good hygiene regarding pet feces
  - Deworming of pets
  - Handwashing after contact with pets, soil, sandboxes, playgrounds
  - Avoiding undercooked meat
- Albendazole 400 mg PO (BID for adults, QD for children) for 5 days
  - Prolonged treatment may lead to pancytopenia
- Mebendazole 100–200 mg BID for 5 days (both pediatric and adult)
  - Only available in the United States through compounding pharmacies
  - Albendazole is preferred in ocular toxocariasis, as it crosses the blood–brain barrier
- Topical and systemic corticosteroids are given along with systemic anthelmintic therapy to address active ocular inflammation
- Vitrectomy for vitreoretinal complications such as epiretinal membrane and retinal detachment

Referral/Co-management

- Infectious Disease
- Pulmonology
- Gastroenterology
- Cardiology
- Neurology

Ascariasis

52

Overview

- Definition
  - Helminthic infection caused by nematode *Ascaris lumbricoides*
  - Acquired by ingestion of embryonated eggs
  - Larvae pass through pulmonary migration phase for maturation
    Typically reside in the jejunum
- Symptoms
  - Often asymptomatic
  - May have redness, irritation, blurring
- Laterality
  - Unilateral
- Course
  - Subacute, rare
- Age of onset
  - Mostly toddlers to adolescents; peak incidence between 2 and 14 years
- Gender/race
  - No gender or racial predilection
  - More prevalent in crowded rural areas, decreased sanitation
  - Highly endemic in China, India, Southeast Asia, Africa, Latin America
- Systemic association
  - Pulmonary, intestinal, peritoneal, hepatobiliary, pancreatic ascariasis
  - Infected youth may develop protein deficiency, malnutrition, growth retardation, intestinal obstruction, perforation, or volvulus, reduced cognitive function

C. S. Foster et al. (eds.), *Uveitis*, https://doi.org/10.1007/978-3-030-52974-1_52

Exam: Ocular

Anterior Segment

- Anterior uveitis
- Nasolacrimal infestation

Posterior Segment

- Visceral larva migrans reported, but controversial

Exam: Systemic

- Often asymptomatic unless heavy wormload
- Self-limiting pneumonia for 2–3 weeks, occurring 4–16 days after ingesting eggs
  - Sudden onset of significant URI symptoms, fever, cough, wheeze
  - Hemoptysis in severe cases
- Vague abdominal pain, distention, nausea, occasional diarrhea
- Peritonitis – may be fatal
- Hepatobiliary or pancreatic involvement

Imaging

- n/a

Laboratory and Radiographic Testing

- Sputum, vomitus, or stool samples show eggs or adult worm
- CBC with differential – high eosinophilia (>10%) common
- Radiology
  - Chest – diffuse, mottled pulmonary infiltrate
  - Abdominal with barium contrast – sharply outlined radiolucency
    Barium inside worm shows filamentous radio-opacity
- Ultrasound – biliary and pancreatic (4-line sign)
- ERCP – smooth, linear filling defects
- Diagnostic vitrectomy (may be therapeutic)

Differential Diagnosis

- Rare, must have high suspicion
- Any cause of anterior uveitis

Treatment

- Pyrantel pamoate 10 mg/kg PO, single dose
  - Contraindicated in hepatic disease, pregnancy
- Mebendazole 100 mg PO BID × 3 days – treatment of choice
  - Contraindicated in pregnancy
- Albendazole 400 mg PO, single dose
  - Contraindicated in pregnancy

Referral/Co-management

- Primary Care
- Infectious Disease
- Pulmonology
- Gastroenterology

Onchocerciasis

53

Overview

- Definition
  - Commonly known as "river blindness," this eye and skin disease is caused by filaria (worm) *Onchocerca volvulus*, transmitted by female *Simulium* blackfly, which breeds in fast-flowing rivers
  - Second to trachoma as the most common infectious cause of blindness worldwide: >15 million people infected
- Symptoms
  - Photophobia, tearing, foreign body sensation
  - Decreased vision
  - Visual field constriction
  - Nyctalopia
- Laterality
  - Bilateral and symmetric
- Course
  - Several years may separate initial infection and clinical presentation
  - Untreated disease results in blindness
- Age of onset
  - Rare in children and teenagers, but increases in the third decade due to rising microfilarial load
- Gender/race
  - Males more commonly affected due to outdoor responsibilities
  - Most common in equatorial Africa, but also in Central/South America and Eastern Mediterranean
- Systemic association
  - Skin disease
  - 20% of patients are co-infected with *Loa Loa* (Chap. 54), a fact bearing significant treatment implications

C. S. Foster et al. (eds.), *Uveitis*, https://doi.org/10.1007/978-3-030-52974-1_53

Exam: Ocular

Skin and eye diseases are caused by microfilaria (offspring) and not macrofilaria (mother). Ocular disease develops due to dead microfilariae, as living microfilariae are, in fact, well tolerated in the eye.

Anterior Segment

- Conjunctivitis and 0.5- to 2-mm diameter conjunctival nodules
- Limbal edema and hyperemia
- Dead microfilariae can be seen directly in the cornea, appearing straight and opaque
- Punctate or sclerosing keratitis
- Anterior uveitis is rare and does not correlate with microfilaria load, and varies from low-grade, non-granulomatous to severe, turbid, granulomatous
- Pupillary seclusion leading to angle closure glaucoma
- Cataract

Posterior Segment

- Pigment clumping and RPE atrophy, either diffuse or geographic with distinct borders, located temporal to the macula or nasal to the optic nerve
- Cotton wool spots and intraretinal hemorrhage
- Intraretinal worms can be seen as reflective opacities with green tint
- Vascular sheathing
- Optic neuritis resulting in optic atrophy and peripapillary hyperpigmentation

Exam: Systemic

- Dermatitis papules is most common with pruritus at acute stage
- Pretibial skin depigmentation ("leopard skin")
- Chronic disease results in skin lichenification and scarring, atrophy, pigment changes, especially on buttocks, waist, shoulders
- Facial skin eruption and purplish lesions on upper body are rare but seen in Central America
- Groups of round, painless, subcutaneous nodules with firm fibrous capsule containing adult worms (15–40 mm, lifespan 10 years)
- Lymphatic obstruction with microfilariae, generally inguinal or femoral

Imaging

- FA: mottled fluorescence around RPE atrophy
- Visual field: diffuse constriction

Laboratory and Radiographic Testing

- Sensitive, low-cost detection of antigens in tears, urine, dermal fluid
- PCR assay with superficial skin scratch, or microscopic skin snip evaluation
- Ultrasonography to detect and evaluate nodules
- ELISA and radioimmunoassay test for parasite specific antibodies

Differential Diagnosis

- Contact dermatitis
- Scabies
- Prickly heat
- Insect bites
- Leprosy, yaws, or superficial mycosis
- Nodule differentiation from lymph node, lipoma, fibroma, dermal cyst, ganglia

Treatment

- Ivermectin is the treatment of choice
  - Kills microfilariae but not macrofilariae
  - Given at 150 mcg/kg in one oral dose every 6–12 months, both adults and children
  - Length of treatment depends on disease activity (continuous skin manifestation is a good gauge) and whether the patient still lives in endemic areas
  - However, serious and sometimes fatal adverse reactions occur in those co-infected with loiasis
- Doxycycline is emerging as a treatment to kill or sterilize macrofilariae
  - Kills *Wolbachia*, an endosymbiotic bacteria required for the survival of *O. volvulus* macrofilariae and embryogenesis
  - Given at 200 mg PO QD for 6 weeks
  - Since it does not kill microfilariae, ivermectin may still need to be given to reduce symptoms
  - Limited data suggest it may be safe in loiasis co-infection
- Topical corticosteroids and cycloplegia to reduce ocular inflammation and positive pupillary seclusion and resultant angle closure glaucoma

Referral/Co-management

- Dermatology and/or Interventional Radiology for nodulectomy

Loiasis

54

Overview

- Definition
  - Chronic infection caused by the filarial parasite *Loa loa*
    Endemic to Africa, but now more widespread owing to travel
  - Humans are only known reservoirs; contracted by bites of *Chrysops* tabanid flies
  - Microfilariae, larvae, and adult worms travel via lymphatics to various organ systems
- Symptoms
  - Blurring
  - Redness
  - Irritation
  - May be asymptomatic
- Laterality
  - Typically unilateral
- Course
  - Chronic, may take months to become symptomatic
- Age of onset
  - All age groups affected
- Gender/race
  - No gender or racial predilection
  - Occur more often in individuals in endemic areas
- Systemic association
  - Calabar swellings, angioedema
  - Also nephropathy, cardiomyopathy, arthritis, lymphangitis, peripheral neuropathy, encephalopathy

C. S. Foster et al. (eds.), *Uveitis*, https://doi.org/10.1007/978-3-030-52974-1_54

Exam: Ocular

Anterior Segment

- Adult worm presenting subconjunctival or in anterior chamber
  - Conjunctival nodules (dead worm)
  - Adult moving worm (most common)
  - Anterior uveitis
  - Fibrous membrane in angle
  - Edema of iris or ciliary body
  - Cataract
  - Ocular hypertension

Posterior Segment

- Microfilariae presenting subretinal, retinal vascular, or choroidal
  - Perivascular inflammatory infiltrate
  - Retinal edema
  - Exudative retinal detachment
  - Vascular or microaneurysm occlusion
  - Large hemorrhagic sheets

Exam: Systemic

- Calabar swellings
  - Localized areas of erythema and angioedema 5–10 cm in size
  - Usually on extremities, joints, spontaneous regression, and reappearance
  - May also have pruritic, vesicular rash
- Nephropathy – proteinuria, chronic glomerulonephritis
- Encephalopathy increasingly common
  - Insomnia, irritability, depression, headache, coma, and death
- Allergic and angioedema symptoms are more prevalent in those who are visiting endemic areas

Imaging

- OCT: subretinal fluid or choroidal thickening

Laboratory and Radiographic Testing

- Collect specimen, between 10 a.m. and 2 p.m.

- Serum eosinophilia
- Elevated anti-filarial antibody
- PCR

Differential Diagnosis

- Cutaneous larval migrans
- Onchocerciasis
- Myiasis
- Cysticercosis

Treatment

- Surgical removal of worm
  - Topical anesthetic (10% cocaine or atropine, never pilocarpine)
  - Incise conjunctiva and firm removal with forceps
- Extermination of microfilariae and other worms
  - Diethylcarbamazine (DEC)
    - Target dose 6–8 mg/kg divided TID for 3 weeks
    - Add 50 mg daily until target
    - Life-threatening adverse reactions (50%) following treatment
    - With high microfilarial load (>30,000/mL), gradual dosing with corticosteroids
  - Ivermectin 50–200 mcg/kg
    - Safer but not effective vs. adult worms
    - Pretreatment for DEC
  - Albendazole 200 mg BID x 3 weeks
    - Only effective vs. adult worms
- Prophylaxis
  - DEC 300 mg PO weekly or DEC 200 mg BID × 3 consecutive days/month

Referral/Co-management

- Primary Care
- Infectious Disease
- Nephrology
- Neurology
- Cardiology

Cysticercosis

55

Overview

- Definition
  - Parasitic infection caused by larval cysts of pork tapeworm *Taenia solium*, affecting the brain, eyes, and muscles
  - A person contracts cysticercosis by ingesting eggs found in the feces of a person with the intestinal tapeworm (via contaminated vegetables or water); it is *not* contracted by eating undercooked pork
  - Can be asymptomatic for months to years; signs and symptoms occur when cysts begin to die, leading to localized swelling and inflammation
  - Ocular disease affects 13–46% of cysticercosis patients and may affect the orbit, adnexa, and intraocular contents
- Symptoms
  - Orbital disease: diplopia, periocular swelling and pain
  - Ocular disease: painful swelling of conjunctiva, floaters, blurry vision
- Laterality
  - Unilateral and unifocal; bilateral and unilateral multifocal cases are very rare
- Course
  - Cysts can be asymptomatic for years but worsen acutely when they begin to die
- Age of onset
  - 10–30 years
- Gender/race
  - No gender predilection
  - Common in countries with poor sanitation in Central and South America, Mexico, sub-Saharan Africa, the Indian subcontinent, and Southeast Asia
- Systemic association
  - Neurocysticercosis
    - Seizures, headaches, confusion, loss of balance
    - Most common cause of adult seizures in low-income countries
    - Can result in death

C. S. Foster et al. (eds.), *Uveitis*, https://doi.org/10.1007/978-3-030-52974-1_55

Exam: Ocular

Orbit and Adnexa

- Lid swelling and ptosis
- Proptosis
- Ocular motility restriction
- Subconjunctival cysts with injection

Anterior Segment

- Mild-to-moderate anterior uveitis
- Translucent white cyst with invaginated scolex (front of the worm)
- Clear lens

Posterior Segment

- Cysts much more common than anterior segment (vitreous > retinal/subretinal)
- Mild to severe vitritis
- Posterior pole hemorrhage and exudates
- Rhegmatogenous or exudative retinal detachment
- Optic disc edema or atrophy

Exam: Systemic

- Change in mental status
- Tender subcutaneous lumps representing muscle cysts

Imaging

- Ultrasonography: Brightness scan (B-scan) shows a well-defined cyst with a hyperechoic center representing the scolex (anterior end of the worm); amplitude scan (A-scan) shows high-amplitude spikes corresponding to the cyst wall and the scolex

Laboratory and Radiographic Testing

- MRI and CT of the orbits: crucial in detecting orbital cysticercosis, seen as a hypodense mass with a central hyperdense scolex
- Stool examination for adult worms

- Anti-cysticercus antibodies not always detectable via ELISA in mild infection. Serologies are only supportive

Differential Diagnosis

- Focal active necrotizing chorioretinitis or retinochoroiditis
- Causes of retrolental white mass or leukocoria: retinoblastoma, Coats disease, retinopathy of prematurity, persistent fetal vasculature, retinal detachment
- Diffuse unilateral subacute neuroretinitis (DUSN)

Treatment

- Combination therapy of oral albendazole (praziquantel is less effective) and corticosteroids is superior to surgical excision in extraocular cysticercosis but generally not effective in intraocular disease
- Posterior segment cysticercosis can lead to blindness and phthisis bulbi if left untreated within 3–5 years
- Destruction of larva less than 8 mm can be done by diathermy, photocoagulation, or cryotherapy; destruction of larva 8 mm or larger without concurrent surgical removal, however, results in extensive inflammatory reaction leading to blindness and phthisis bulbi
- Early surgical larva removal is the definitive therapy for intraocular cysticercosis; PPV with retinotomy is preferred over external approach with posterior sclerotomy, as the latter is associated with a high complication rate

Referral/Co-management

- Infectious Disease
- Neurology

Diffuse Unilateral Subacute Neuroretinitis

56

Overview

- Definition
  - Progressive disease involving outer retina and RPE, caused by nematode larvae: *Toxocara canis*, *Baylisacaris procyonis* (Midwestern United States) and *Ancylostoma caninum* (Southeastern United States, South America), among others
- Symptoms
  - Vision loss
  - Floaters
  - Nyctalopia
  - Pain and photophobia rare
- Laterality
  - Unilateral
  - A few bilateral cases reports
- Course
  - Left untreated, disease progresses and vision rendered 20/400 or worse
- Age of onset
  - Young, with an average of 12 years
- Gender/race
  - No gender or racial predilection
- Systemic association
  - None

C. S. Foster et al. (eds.), *Uveitis*, https://doi.org/10.1007/978-3-030-52974-1_56

Exam: Ocular

Anterior Segment

- APD in all stages
- Conjunctival hyperemia a common early sign
- No AC inflammation
- Cornea and lens not affected

Posterior Segment

- Small, white, motile worm often subretinal, but may be in mid-vitreous or within retina
- Curvilinear marks in RPE = "worm tracks"
- Mild-to-moderate vitritis
- Blurred optic disc margin
- Multiple, focal grayish lesions, about 1 disc diameter in size, in deep retinal layers (immune response to worm) with possible overlying serous retinal detachment; lesions generally not foveal
- Late disease characterized by diffuse pigmentary atrophy, retinal vascular attenuation, and optic atrophy. Severe cases known as "Unilateral Wipe Out" Syndrome.

Exam: Systemic

- N/A

Imaging

- FA
  - Early disease: Hypofluorescence of focal lesions followed by staining; leakage at the optic disc
  - Late disease: Increased retinal circulation time with diffuse, widespread hyperfluorescence; focal window defects at scars
- ICG: Hypocyanescence underlying lesions
- ERG: Mild decrease in rod and cone function, shows decreased B wave

Laboratory and Radiographic Testing

- Eosinophil level only if systemic parasitic spread is suspected

Differential Diagnosis

- Multifocal choroiditis and panuveitis (bilateral)
- APMPPE (bilateral)
- Sarcoidosis
- Toxoplasmosis
- Histoplasmosis
- Occlusive retinal vascular disease
- Post-traumatic chorioretinopathy
- Toxic retinopathy

Treatment

- Photocoagulation of identified nematode
  - If worm is close to fovea, use light laser to "chase" worm into periphery, then destroy with higher power
  - Pars plana vitrectomy to remove worm if laser fails
- If worm is invisible, antihelminthic therapy (albendazole 400 mg/d for 1 month) along with oral prednisone may be considered

Referral/Co-management

- Infectious Disease

57 Schistosomiasis

Overview

- Definition
  - A tropical parasitic disease caused by flatworms of genus *Schistomsomes*, carried by freshwater snails
  - Also known as "snail fever" or "bilharzia"
  - Infection is contracted via skin contact with contaminated freshwater, and disease results from inflammatory reaction to worm eggs that are lodged in the intestine or bladder
  - Affecting 200+ million people worldwide, it is second only to malaria in economic impact in the tropics
- Symptoms
  - Redness
  - Pain
  - Photophobia
  - Blurry vision
- Laterality
  - Often bilateral
- Course
  - Systemic symptoms appear within 1–2 months of infection
  - If untreated, chronic disease can persist for years
  - Ocular granulomas are associated with progressive scarring; choroidal granuloma near the macula results in severe visual loss
- Age of onset
  - All age groups affected
- Gender/race
  - No gender predilection
  - Distributed throughout Africa; areas of the Middle East, South America, Indonesia, China, and Southeast Asia

C. S. Foster et al. (eds.), *Uveitis*, https://doi.org/10.1007/978-3-030-52974-1_57

  - Not found in the United States
- Systemic association
  - Intestinal schistosomiasis (*S. mansoni*, *S. japonicum*, *S. mekongi*, *S. intercalatum*)

    Acute
    - Katayama syndrome: fever, fatigue, malaise, muscle aches, dry cough, abdominal pain, hepatosplenomegaly
    - Diarrhea
    - Bloody stool

    Chronic
    - Cirrhosis and portal hypertension
    - Bowel wall ulceration, hyperplasia, and polyposis
  - Urogenital schistosomiasis (*S. haematobium*)

    Acute
    - Dysuria
    - Hematuria

    Chronic
    - Increased risk of bladder cancer
    - Damage to the vagina, cervix, and fallopian tubes increase susceptibility to other infections
  - CNS disease

    Rare, but can lead to seizures, paralysis, and transverse myelitis

Exam: Ocular

External

- Lid and lacrimal gland granulomas

Anterior Segment

- Subconjunctival granuloma presents as a tender nodule
- Granulomas in the angle structure, which can lead to ocular hypertension

Posterior Segment

- Multiple choroidal granulomas in different stages of pigmentation
- Retinal and choroidal vasculitis
- Neuroretinitis

Exam: Systemic

- Hepatosplenomegaly (intestinal form)
- Vaginal bleeding, nodules in the vulva (urogenital form)

Imaging

- OCT
  - Highly reflective lesions in the choroid
- FA
  - Early hypofluorescence followed by late leakage of retinal/subretinal/choroidal granulomas
- ICG
  - Early hypofluorescence of choroidal lesions that persist into late phase

Laboratory and Radiographic Testing

- Examination for parasitic eggs in urine or stool
  - Samples collected on different days increase sensitivity
- Serologic testing for antischistosomal antibodies
  - Collected at least 6–8 weeks after infection
  - Does not distinguish active vs. treated infection
- Eosinophilia is present with hepatomegaly and/or splenomegaly

Differential Diagnosis

- Sarcoidosis
- Tuberculosis
- Multifocal choroiditis
- APMPPE

Treatment

- Praziquantel
  - 20 mg/kg BID or TID for just 1 day is often curative
  - Given 6–8 weeks after last contact with contaminated freshwater, as the drug is most effective against adult worms
  - Safe in young children and pregnant women
- Topical and systemic corticosteroids for ocular inflammation

Referral/Co-management

- Infectious Disease
- Gastroenterology
- Urology
- Ob-Gyn

Ophthalmomyiasis

58

Overview

- Definition
  - Ocular infestation involving obligate parasitic botfly larvae (order *Diptera)* via direct inoculation
    - Ophthalmomyiasis externa – eyelid and adnexa
    - Ophthalmomyiasis interna – intraocular (rare)
  - Requires animals (sheep, cows, rabbits or rodents) as hosts to complete developmental cycle, and larvae are subsequently passed to humans most commonly via the conjunctival surface directly
  - Larvae mouth hooks and thorax spines result in mechanical injury to eye
  - Can migrate throughout anterior and posterior structures, may avoid examination light
  - Death of parasite can result in ocular inflammation
- Symptoms
  - Tearing
  - Eyelid twitch
  - Irritation
  - Redness
  - Mild blurring
- Laterality
  - Unilateral
- Course
  - Indolent
- Age of onset
  - All age groups affected
- Gender/race
  - No gender or racial predilection
  - Worldwide

C. S. Foster et al. (eds.), *Uveitis*, https://doi.org/10.1007/978-3-030-52974-1_58

- Systemic association
  - None

Exam: Ocular

Anterior Segment

- Motile larvae often seen on conjunctival cul-de-sac or cornea
- Conjunctivitis – Hyperemic with hemorrhages, and follicles
- Keratitis

Posterior Segment

- Direct visualization of larvae
- Subretinal tracks where larvae have traveled
- Vitreous hemorrhage
- Retinal detachment
- Endophthalmitis (rare)
  - Chorioretinitis, purulent panuveitis (usually results from death of larvae)

Exam: Systemic

- None

Imaging

- FA: reveals extent of mechanical injury to RPE and macula via window defects, scarring
- OCT: Intraretinal and subretinal tunnels can be visualized Fundus Photo: White lines often present to show path of tunnels

Laboratory and Radiographic Testing

- Examine removed maggot in fixative to identify species

Differential Diagnosis

- Diffuse unilateral subacute neuroretinitis (DUSN)
- Angioid streaks
- Traumatic choroidal ruptures
- Histoplasmosis

Treatment

- Remove larvae from the ocular surface at slit lamp with topical anesthetic, immobilizing maggot
- Curative and definitive treatment is surgical removal from internal ocular structures
  - Argon laser to kill maggot, but parasite still needs removal via pars plana vitrectomy to avoid inflammatory reaction
- Topical and oral steroids to control inflammation

Referral/Co-management

- Infectious Disease

Ophthalmia Nodosa

59

Overview

- Definition
  - Ocular inflammation due to contact or penetration by hairs or setae of certain insects (e.g., caterpillars) and vegetables
  - Five types

    Type 1 – acute, anaphylactoid reaction consisting of conjunctival chemosis, inflammation, epiphora, and foreign body sensation

    Type 2 – chronic mechanical keratoconjunctivitis caused by hairs lodged in bulbar/palpebral conjunctiva; linear scratches on cornea

    Type 3 – formation of grayish-yellow asymptomatic conjunctival nodules

    Type 4 – intense anterior uveitis due to hair penetration in anterior chamber; often associated with iris nodules and hypopyon

    Type 5 – hair penetration into the vitreous and subretinal space; chorioretinal tracks pigmented with white, inflamed leading edge
  - Patients may develop some or all of the above features sequentially as hairs/setae migrate inwards, though most fall in types 1 and 2
- Symptoms
  - Redness
  - Photophobia
  - Foreign body sensation
  - Blurry vision
  - Floaters
- Laterality
  - Unilateral or bilateral
- Course

  Severity depends on the amount of hairs involved, but long-term prognosis is good in most cases.
  - Type 1: acute and lasts for weeks

C. S. Foster et al. (eds.), *Uveitis*, https://doi.org/10.1007/978-3-030-52974-1_59

  - Type 2: chronic
  - Type 3: asymptomatic
  - Type 4: acute and severe
  - Type 5: may occur early or years after penetration
- Age of onset
  - All age groups affected
- Gender/race
  - No gender or racial predilection
- Systemic association
  - None

Exam: Ocular

Findings vary based on location of foreign materials

Anterior Segment

- Chemosis (type 1)
- Vertical abrasions of corneal epithelium: lid eversion reveals hair as dark spot with surrounding hyperemia near lid margin (type 2)
- Conjunctival nodule (type 3)
- Ciliary flush, anterior chamber inflammation, possible hypopyon, and iris nodules: hair visible in corneal stroma, iris, and adjacent trabecular band, or lens (type 4)

Posterior Segment (Type 5)

- Setae/hairs in cortical vitreous
- Mild-to-moderate vitritis
- Snowballs/snowbanks
- Yellow patches of retinochoroiditis (usually temporal macular area)
- Macular edema
- Papillitis

Exam: Systemic

- Allergic dermatitis

Imaging

- Ultrasound Biomicroscopy (UBM)
  - Setae/hairs appear hyper-reflective
  - Localized swelling of iris and ciliary body

Laboratory and Radiographic Testing

- None

Differential Diagnosis

- Diffuse unilateral subacute neuroretinitis (DUSN)
- Penetrating injury by other foreign materials

Treatment

- Type 1: copious irrigation and topical steroids
- Type 2: removal of hairs by forceps with lid eversion
- Type 3: removal of conjunctival nodules (to prevent migration to cornea and subsequently other intraocular structures)
- Type 4: topical steroids for keratitis and anterior uveitis; removal of hairs with forceps, iridectomy, and even lensectomy; neodymium:yttrium-aluminum-garnet (Nd:YAG) laser to disrupt hairs
- Type 5: oral, periocular, or intraocular steroids for inflammatory control (but other infections must be ruled out before ocular injections); Nd:YAG laser to disrupt hairs; vitrectomy for resistant cases

Referral/Co-management

- None

HIV-Associated Uveitis

60

HIV (Human Immunodeficiency Virus)

Overview

- Retrovirus that infects $CD4^+$ T lymphocyte (cell-mediated immunity)
- Severe immunodeficiency permits the development of opportunistic infections and malignancies
- Transmission
  - Sexual contact
  - Blood: Intravenous Drug Use (IVDU), blood products
  - Mother to child
- Highly active antiretroviral therapy (HAART) has led to dramatic improvement in the prognosis of HIV infection

Ocular Manifestations of HIV Infection

- Most common
  - Ocular manifestation of human immunodeficiency virus, acquired immunodeficiency syndrome (HIV-AIDS): HIV retinopathy
  - Retinal opportunistic infection: Cytomegalovirus (CMV) retinitis
- Multifocal choroiditis
  - Tuberculosis (TB), mycobacterium avium complex, histoplasmosis, cryptococcosis, pneumocystosis, other fungi, lymphoma
  - Look for disseminated systemic infection

C. S. Foster et al. (eds.), *Uveitis*, https://doi.org/10.1007/978-3-030-52974-1_60

HIV Retinopathy

Overview

- Definition
  - Retinal microvasculopathy
  - Most common ocular manifestation of HIV-AIDS
- Symptoms
  - Asymptomatic
  - Blurring with macular involvement
- Laterality: Mostly bilateral
- Course: Spontaneously resolved within weeks or months
- Age of onset: any
- Gender/race: no gender or racial predilection
- Systemic association: Usually found in HIV patients with low CD4 count

Exam: Ocular

Anterior Segment

- No inflammation

Posterior Segment

- Cotton-wool spots
  - Posterior pole, often adjacent to retinal vessels
  - Large or progressive lesions should cause suspicion of early CMV retinitis
- Scattered dot blot or flame-shaped hemorrhages
- Microaneurysms
- Isolated perivascular sheathing without opportunistic infections
  - Common in African patients (especially children)

Exam: Systemic

- Variable depending on opportunistic infections
- Acute systemic infection (HIV prodrome)
  - Occurs days to weeks after inoculation
  - Fever, lymphadenopathy, pharyngitis, rash, myalgia, malaise, headache, nausea, weight loss, diarrhea, night sweats, neurologic symptoms
  - Patients are more infectious during acute primary infection
- Latent stage
  - Occurs weeks to years after inoculation
  - Lymphadenopathy

- Acquired immune deficiency syndrome (AIDS)
  - Less common in the setting of HAART
  - Designated as AIDS with the onset of opportunistic infections or malignancies that are uncommon in the general population

Imaging

- FA: hyperfluorescent microaneurysms; microvasculopathy, occlusive disease; blocking defects with hemorrhages

Laboratory and Radiographic Testing

- HIV 1/2 Ag Ab immunoassay
- CD4 count/%
- Viral load
- Complete Blood Count (CBC) with differential
- Comprehensive Metabolic Panel (CMP)
- βhCG
- Serologic screening for various infectious comorbidities

Differential Diagnosis

- Early CMV retinopathy
- Diabetes/hypertensive retinopathy

Treatment

- No treatment for HIV retinopathy
- HAART for systemic infection

Referral/Co-management

- Infectious Disease
- Primary Care

CMV Retinitis

See Chap. 35 Herpesviruses

Immune Recovery Uveitis (IRU)

Overview

- Definition
  - An ocular form of immune reconstitution inflammatory syndrome (IRIS) involving increased ocular inflammation in previously opportunistic infected eyes, after improvement of immune function from HAART therapy
    - CMV (most common)
    - TB
    - *Toxoplasma*
  - Typically manifests 2–16 weeks after CD4 count increases above 100 cells/μL following the initiation of HAART
- Symptoms
  - Asymptomatic
  - Blurring
  - Floaters
- Laterality: unilateral or bilateral
- Course: subacute
- Age of onset: any
- Gender/race: no gender or racial predilection; any exposed individual
- Systemic association
  - Diseases associated
    - CMV retinitis: most common
    - Inactive toxoplasmosis
    - Tuberculous retinochoroiditis
    - Cryptococcal infection
  - Risk factors
    - Inactive CMV retinitis involving more than 30% of retinal area
    - Patients initially treated with cidofovir
    - Low $CD4^{+}$ cell before starting HAART

Exam: Ocular

Anterior Segment

- Anterior uveitis
- Cataract

Posterior Segment

- Vitritis
- Cystoid macular edema (CME)
- Epiretinal membrane
- Retinal and optic disc neovascularization
- Glaucoma

Exam: Systemic

- Variable depending on opportunistic infections
- Same as HIV retinopathy, but expect systemic course to be improved with immune recovery

Imaging

- OCT: CME, ERM

Laboratory and Radiographic Testing

- CD4 count elevated above 100 cells/μL
- Serologic testing to evaluate for/rule out other forms of inflammation

Differential Diagnosis

- Relapse of the previous infection
- New opportunistic infection

Treatment

- Can be self-limiting
- Appropriate antimicrobial therapy
- Topical corticosteroid for anterior segment inflammation
- Mild vitritis without CME with good vision can be observed
- Intravitreal, periocular, or short-course systemic corticosteroids for vitritis and CME

Pneumocystis carinii Choroidopathy

Overview

- Definition
  - Caused by fungus *Pneumocystis jirovecii* (former name *Pneumocystis carinii*)
  - Choroidal involvement is a sign of disseminated life-threatening fungal infection
- Symptoms
  - Loss of central vision or no visual disturbance
- Laterality: mostly bilateral

- Course: subacute
- Age of onset: any
- Gender/race: no predilection; any exposed individual
- Systemic association
  - CD4 count below 50 cells/μL (in contrast to CD4 200 cells/μL in pneumonia patient)
  - Pulmonary infection
  - Extrapulmonary: lymph nodes, spleen, liver, bone marrow

Exam: Ocular

Anterior Segment

- No anterior chamber reaction

Posterior Segment

- Plaque-like, deep, yellow-white, round or multilobular foci at the posterior pole
- No vitritis or vasculitis

Exam: Systemic

- Full physical examination may reveal findings, especially in lung, lymph nodes, and GI

Imaging

- FA: early hypofluorescence and late staining

Laboratory and Radiographic Testing

- Diagnosis is based on clinical and FA findings
- Systemic workup for disseminated disease: Chest X-ray, sputum culture, CBC, liver function test

Differential Diagnosis

- Fungus: candidiasis, cryptococcosis, histoplasmosis
- Syphilis
- Tuberculosis, mycobacterium avium complex
- Primary intraocular lymphoma

Treatment

- Systemic trimetroprim (15 mg/kg/day)–sulfamethoxazole (75 mg/kg/day) in 3 divided doses, for 21 days
- Followed by secondary prophylaxis until immune reconstitution (CD4 >200 cells/μL)

Referral/Co-management

- Infectious Disease
- Pulmonologist

Mycobacterium Avium Complex (MAC)

Overview

- Definition
  - MAC disease typically is a disseminated, multi-organ infection in AIDS patients who are not on HAART.
  - The mode of transmission: inhalation, ingestion, or inoculation via the respiratory or gastrointestinal tract.
- Symptoms
  - Blurring
  - Floaters
- Laterality: unilateral, but bilateral can occur
- Course: subacute
- Age of onset: any
- Gender/race: no gender or racial predilection; any exposed individual
- Systemic association
  - CD4 T cells <50 cells/μL
  - Fever, night sweats, weight loss, diarrhea, anemia, and abdominal pain

Exam: Ocular

Anterior Segment

- Granulomatous anterior uveitis
- Iris nodules

Posterior Segment

- Multifocal choroiditis with panuveitis
- Unifocal choroidal infiltrate
- Endophthalmitis

Exam: Systemic

- Hepatomegaly, splenomegaly, lymphadenopathy, and skin lesion

Laboratory and Radiographic Testing

- Ocular fluid or tissue
  - Gram, modified Acid fast bacilli (AFB), AFB staining
  - Culture and PCR for mycobacterium
- CBC, liver function test, chest X-ray

Differential Diagnosis

- Fungus: candidiasis, cryptococcosis, histoplasmosis, pneumocystosis
- Syphilis
- TB
- Intraocular lymphoma

Treatment

- At least two antimycobacterial drugs to prevent or delay the emergence of resistance
  - Azithromycin (500 mg daily) or clarithromycin (500 mg PO twice daily) and ethambutol (15 mg/kg PO daily)
- Alternative therapy: rifabutin (300 mg PO daily), levofloxacin (500 mg PO daily), moxifloxacin (400 mg PO daily), amikacin, streptomycin
- Followed by secondary prophylaxis until immune reconstitution (CD4 >100 cells/μL) and disease controlled

Referral/Co-management

- Infectious disease

Endophthalmitis

61

Chronic Postoperative Endophthalmitis

Overview

- Definition
  - Recurrent episodes of inflammation due to microbes introduced during intraocular surgery:
    - Chronic endophthalmitis occurs >1 month after surgery
    - Acute endophthalmitis occurs <1 month after surgery
- Symptoms
  - Blurry vision
  - Photophobia
  - Redness
- Laterality
  - Unilateral (postsurgical eye only)
- Course
  - Recurrent episodes of indolent, chronic inflammation occur weeks, months, or years after intraocular surgery (typically after cataract surgery)
    - Bacterial endophthalmitis improves with steroids, worsens on steroid taper
      - *P. acnes* may worsen after Nd:YAG posterior capsulotomy
    - Fungal endophthalmitis worsens with steroids
- Age of onset
  - Not applicable
- Gender/race
  - Not applicable
- Systemic association
  - Silicone lens or lenticular capsular rupture may facilitate ingress of microbes
  - Ocular wound abnormalities increase risk

C. S. Foster et al. (eds.), *Uveitis*, https://doi.org/10.1007/978-3-030-52974-1_61

Exam: Ocular

Anterior Segment

- White "plaque" on lens or posterior capsule (especially *P. acnes*)
- Granulomatous keratic precipitates
- Corneal decompensation
- Iris neovascularization
- Necrotizing scleritis (especially fungal)
- "Fluff balls" in the anterior chamber (especially fungal)

Posterior Segment

- Vitritis
- Snowballs
- "String-of-pearls" vitreous exudate (especially fungal)
- Vascular occlusion with retinal hemorrhages

Exam: Systemic

- None

Imaging

- Ultrasound biomicroscopy (UBM)
  - Bacterial: plaque between IOL and posterior capsule
  - Fungal: iris or ciliary body mass, "fungus ball"

Laboratory and Radiographic Testing

- Send undiluted vitreous fluid or aqueous humor for the following:
  - Aerobic, anaerobic, and fungal culture
  - Gram and Giemsa stains
  - Polymerase chain reaction

Differential Diagnosis

- Granulomatous anterior or panuveitis
- Lens-induced uveitis
- Intraocular lymphoma (especially in elderly patients)
- Uveitis-glaucoma-hyphema syndrome
- Intraocular lens malposition
- Sterile endophthalmitis
- Sympathetic ophthalmia

Treatment

- Pars plana vitrectomy and/or anterior chamber paracentesis
  - Bacterial: intravitreal vancomycin and ceftazidime
  - Fungal: intravitreal voriconazole or amphotericin
    ± systemic and/or topical antifungals
- If recalcitrant: intraocular lens explant with capsulectomy

Referral/Comanagement

- Not applicable

Endogenous Bacterial Endophthalmitis

Overview

- Definition
  - Infection caused by hematogenous spread of bacteria to the eye
- Symptoms
  - Blurry vision
  - Pain
  - Photophobia
- Laterality
  - May be either unilateral or bilateral
- Course
  - Acute, severe onset of symptoms in an immunocompromised patient
    A systemic nidus of infection is found in >90% of cases
- Age of onset
  - All ages
- Gender/Race
  - N/a
- Systemic association
  - Common causative organisms include the following:
    Streptococci (beware of endocarditis)
    Staphylococci
    Enteric pathogens (e.g., *Klebsiella, E. coli*)
    Bacillus cereus (especially among intravenous drug users)
    Encapsulated bacteria (e.g., *H. influenzae*, *N. meningitidis*)
  - Risk factors: diabetes mellitus, HIV, systemic lupus erythematosus, sickle cell disease, intravenous drug abuse, indwelling catheter use, recent gastrointestinal surgery, recent dental procedure, recent hospitalization, acutely ill/septic
  - Common sites of infection include the following:

Subacute bacterial endocarditis
Pneumonia
Gastrointestinal infection
Osteomyelitis
Meningitis
Hepatic abscess

Exam: Ocular

Anterior

- Cells and flare
- Hypopyon
- Iris microabscess
- Chemosis and/or periorbital edema

Posterior

- Vitreous cell/debris
- Roth spots
- Flame-shaped retinal hemorrhages
- Retinal/subretinal abscess

Exam: Systemic

- Fever
- Leukocytosis
- Infected indwelling catheter site

Imaging

- B-scan or UBM if view of fundus is blocked

Laboratory and Radiographic Testing

- Attempts to identify the infectious nidus:
  - Chest X-ray
  - Blood and urine cultures
    Culture of indwelling catheter (as applicable)
  - Lumbar puncture (if there is evidence of meningitis)
  - Transesophageal echocardiography (if concern for endocarditis)
- Analysis of undiluted vitreous or aqueous humor to identify causative organism:
  - Gram stain, bacterial culture (aerobic and anaerobic), PCR

Differential Diagnosis

- Chronic postoperative endophthalmitis
- Endogenous fungal endophthalmitis
- Intraocular foreign body with traumatic endophthalmitis
- Noninfectious posterior or intermediate uveitis
- Toxoplasma retinochoroiditis
- Toxocara retinochoroiditis
- Intraocular lymphoma

Treatment

- Patient should be hospitalized with consultation to the internal medicine and/or infectious disease service
- Intravenous broad-spectrum antibiotics
- Topical corticosteroids with cycloplegia
- Intravitreal antibiotics (vancomycin plus ceftazidime)
- Pars plana vitrectomy in severe cases

Referral/Comanagement

- Infectious disease
- Internal medicine inpatient service

Endogenous Fungal Endophthalmitis

Overview

- Definition
  - Infection caused by hematogenous spread of fungi to the eye
- Symptoms
  - Blurry vision
  - Pain
  - Photophobia
- Laterality
  - Typically bilateral
- Course
  - Acute onset of symptoms, which are typically less severe than endogenous bacterial endophthalmitis and worsen with corticosteroid use
    Begins as a multifocal retinochoroiditis with potential dissemination to the vitreous body
- Age of onset
  - All ages

- Gender/Race
  - n/a
- Systemic association
  - Causative organisms:
    - *Candida albicans* (most common)
    - *Aspergillus* spp.
    - Less common: *Coccidioidomycosis immitis*, *Cryptococcus neoformans*, *Blastomyces dermatitides*, *Sporothrix schenkii*, *Histoplasma capsulatum*
  - All patients with candidemia should have baseline dilated ocular examination within 72 hours of diagnosis and again 2 weeks after diagnosis, even if asymptomatic
  - Risk factors: neutropenia, hyperalimentation, recent gastrointestinal surgery, diabetes mellitus, intravenous drug use, indwelling catheters, acute illness/sepsis, organ transplant, recent neonatal hospitalization

Exam: Ocular

Anterior

- Hypopyon
- Keratic precipitates
- Cells and flare
- Iris nodules
- Rubeosis iridis

Posterior

- Yellow-white multifocal choroiditis
  - Lesions <1 mm in diameter suggest *Candida* spp.
  - Macular lesions suggest *Aspergillus* spp.
- "String-of-pearls" vitreous exudates or "fluff balls" (suggest *Candida* spp.)
- Retinal hemorrhages (suggest *Aspergillus* spp.)
- Chorioretinal ischemia (suggests *Aspergillus* spp.)

Exam: Systemic

- Infected indwelling catheter

Imaging

- B-scan or UBM if view of posterior segment is poor

Laboratory and Radiographic Testing

- Analysis of undiluted vitreous to identify causative organism:
  - Giemsa stain, fungal culture, PCR
    Candida spp.: budding yeast with pseudohyphae
    Aspergillus spp.: septate hyphae that branch at acute angles

Differential Diagnosis

- Noninfectious intermediate or posterior uveitis
- CMV retinitis
- Endogenous bacterial endophthalmitis
- Toxoplasma retinochoroiditis

Treatment

- Hospitalization with consultation to the inpatient internal medicine or infectious disease service
- Ocular candidiasis
  - If there is no vitreal involvement: oral voriconazole 200 mg twice daily for 4 weeks
  - If there is vitritis:
    Pars plana vitrectomy (PPV)
    Intravitreal amphotericin B or voriconazole
  - If there is severe ocular or systemic disease, supplement above with intravenous amphotericin B ± flucytosine
- Other fungal agents, including *Aspergillus* spp.
  - Treat aggressively with PPV, intravitreal antifungals, and intravenous antifungals

Referral/Comanagement

- Infectious disease

62 Vitreoretinal Lymphoma

Overview

- Definition
  - Intraocular lymphoma mimicking intermediate, posterior, or panuveitis in older patients not responsive to steroid therapy; typical subtype is diffuse, large B-cell, non-Hodgkin's
  - Primary intraocular lymphoma (PIOL) denotes absence of central nervous system (CNS) involvement
- Symptoms
  - Blurry vision
  - Floaters
  - Scotoma
  - Frank inflammatory symptoms such as redness, pain, and photophobia are rare unless there is significant anterior segment infiltration
- Laterality
  - 80% bilateral
- Course
  - Insidious and progressive
- Age of onset
  - 50–60 years (range 15–85)
- Gender/race
  - Slight female and Caucasian predilection
- Systemic association: CNS lymphoma
  - 20% of CNS lymphoma patients have ocular disease at the time of diagnosis; however
  - If intraocular lymphoma is diagnosed first, 60–80% develop CNS disease after 2–3 years

C. S. Foster et al. (eds.), *Uveitis*, https://doi.org/10.1007/978-3-030-52974-1_62

- Overall, intraocular-CNS lymphoma makes up only 1% of all non-Hodgkin's lymphoma in immunocompetent patients (200 cases diagnosed a year in the United States)
- Higher incidence of intraocular-CNS lymphoma in acquired immunodeficiency syndrome (AIDS), post-organ transplant, and congenital immunodeficiencies

Exam: Ocular

Anterior Segment

- No or very mild external sign of inflammation
- Conjunctival hyperemia
- Keratic precipitates
- Mild Anterior Chamber reaction

Posterior Segment

- Large clumps or sheets of cells in vitreous
- Mild to very dense vitritis
- Multifocal, large, yellow sub-RPE or subretinal infiltrates

Exam: Systemic

- Headache
- Personality change
- Alertness alteration
- Memory loss
- Nausea/vomiting
- Gait imbalance
- Weakness
- Seizure

Imaging

- OCT: Sub-RPE hyper-reflective material; no CME
- FA: RPE granularity and possible blockage corresponding to sub-RPE infiltrates, but no vasculitis, papillitis, or macular leakage that would be expected in inflammatory syndromes

Laboratory and Radiographic Testing

- Gold standard for ocular diagnosis is either
  - Vitreous biopsy or sub-RPE aspirate via pars plana vitrectomy; not uncommon to need repeat biopsy if first one negative; ALL following analyses are recommended to have best yield
    - Undiluted sample for cytopathology
    - Diluted sample for molecular genetics to look for monoclonality
      - IgH gene rearrangement: B-cell lymphoma
      - T-cell receptor gene rearrangement: T-cell lymphoma
    - Diluted sample for interleukin (IL)-6 and -10 levels
      - High IL-10/6 consistent with lymphoma
  - Chorioretinal biopsy
    - Used when there is obvious, focal chorioretinal lesion but little vitreous cellularity
    - Significantly higher ocular morbidity than vitreous biopsy alone (retinal detachment, vitreous hemorrhage, proliferative vitreoretinopathy, etc.)
- MRI brain to assess extent of any CNS involvement
  - Deep brain structures, especially front lobe, are more often involved than cerebral cortex compared to other brain tumors (thus change in personality and alertness).
  - Supratentorial and multicentric in half the cases; characteristically dense and diffuse enhancement with distinct borders.
- Positron emission tomography (PET) (may not detect Primary intraocular lymphoma [PIOL])
- Lumbar puncture: Required in all patients suspected of CNS lymphoma

Differential Diagnosis

- Sarcoidosis
- Tuberculosis
- White dot syndromes, especially Birdshot
  - White dot syndrome in an older patient → think lymphoma
- Viral retinitis
- Lymphoid hyperplasia of the uvea (usually unilateral and responds well to steroids)
- Amelanotic uveal melanoma
- Uveal metastasis

Treatment

- Local therapies

  - Intravitreal methotrexate (MTX) 400 mcg/0.1 cc or rituximab (RTX) 1 mg/0.1 cc weekly for 6 weeks, extended as needed if cellularity or lesion persists; repeat cycles as needed
  - If subretinal lymphoma is threatening macula and there is little suspicion for infectious uveitis, then empiric intravitreal MTX may be appropriate before biopsy result is available
  - External beam radiation
- Given the high rate of eventual CNS involvement, we recommend systemic chemotherapy as prophylaxis even if there is no CNS involvement at the time of diagnosis

Referral/Co-management

- Neuro-oncology
- Radiation oncology
- Neurology

Ocular Leukemia

63

Overview

- Ocular involvement is a sign of severe disease.
  - May be the first sign of disease relapse
- Most common in children with acute lymphoblastic leukemia
  - Overall, <5% of patients with systemic leukemia have true ocular infiltration

Exam

- Leukemic infiltrates
- Pseudohypopyon, spontaneous hyphema
- Extensive intraretinal hemorrhages
- Cotton wool spots
- Peripheral retinal microaneurysms (especially in chronic leukemia)
- Vitreous hemorrhage
- Optic disc edema or hemorrhage

Imaging

- FA and ultrasonography do not show any specific findings
- Fine needle aspiration or diagnostic pars plana vitrectomy (PPV)
  - Leukemic blast cells

C. S. Foster et al. (eds.), *Uveitis*, https://doi.org/10.1007/978-3-030-52974-1_63

Differential Diagnosis

- Uveitis
- Retinoblastoma
- Endophthalmitis (with opportunistic infection)
- Radiation-induced ophthalmopathy

Treatment

- Systemic chemotherapy
- Ocular radiotherapy (especially for optic nerve involvement)

Ocular Metastasis

64

Overview

- The most common type of ocular malignancy, typically affecting the choroid
- Uveal metastasis most commonly originates in the breast or lung
- Most commonly affects Caucasian females >60 years of age
  - Overall 5-year-survival is <25%, with mean survival of <24 months

Exam

- Symptoms: blurry vision, flashes, and floaters; asymptomatic in 10% of cases
- Commonly presents as a yellow subretinal mass with associated subretinal fluid
  - Typically unilateral, with one to two lesions present
  - Average lesional dimensions: 9 mm in diameter, 3 mm thick

Imaging

- Fundus autofluorescence
  - Tumor hypoautofluorescence with areas of overlying hyperautofluorescence corresponding to lipofuscin and subretinal fluid
- Ultrasonography
  - Amplitude scan (A-scan): Highly reflective mass
  - Brightness scan (B-scan): Hyper-echogenic mass with a low height-to-base ratio
- Ocular coherence tomography (OCT)
  - Subretinal fluid with choroidal undulations ("lumpy bumpy" appearance)

C. S. Foster et al. (eds.), *Uveitis*, https://doi.org/10.1007/978-3-030-52974-1_64

- Fluorescein angiography
  - Early hypofluorescence with late hyperfluorescence
  - Pinpoint leakage at the tumor margin
- Magnetic resonance imaging (MRI)
  - Well-demarcated choroidal mass that is isointense on T1- and hypointense on T2-weighted images

Differential Diagnosis

- Primary uveal melanoma
- Hemangioma
- Granuloma

Treatment

- Systemic chemotherapy
- Plaque radiotherapy
- Transpupillary thermoplasty
- Enucleation for painful eye or observation if prognosis is poor
- Other therapies include: proton beam radiotherapy, gamma knife radiosurgery, external beam radiotherapy, photodynamic therapy, or intravitreal anti-vascular endothelial growth factor (VEGF) injections

Uveal Melanoma

65

Overview

- Definition
  - A malignant melanocytic proliferation within the uveal tract
  - The most common primary intraocular malignancy
- Symptoms
  - Typically asymptomatic
  - Blurry vision, photopsias, floaters, metamorphopsia
- Age of onset
  - 50–60 years
- Gender/race
  - M > F
  - Caucasian > Hispanic > Asian > Black
  - Factors associated with increased host susceptibility include:
    - Light irides, fair skin
    - Oculodermal melanocytosis
    - BRCA1-associated protein 1 (BAP1) mutation
    - GNA Q/11 mutation
- Epidemiology
  - Incidence of 5.1 per million per year in the United States
  - 5% of all melanomas, 83% of all ocular melanomas
  - Choroidal melanoma accounts for 90% of uveal melanomas
  - Prognosis
    - Iris melanoma shows 9% risk of metastasis at 10 years and 3% risk of mortality at 10 years
      - Worse prognosis associated with secondary glaucoma, older age at diagnosis, increased tumor thickness, involvement of iris root or angle structures and extraocular extension

C. S. Foster et al. (eds.), *Uveitis*, https://doi.org/10.1007/978-3-030-52974-1_65

Posterior uveal melanoma has a high rate of metastasis and mortality

- Metastasis to the liver, lung, bone, skin, and lymph nodes
- Worse prognosis is associated with, among other histopathologic and cytogenetic features: increasing age, male gender, large lesion diameter, increased lesional thickness, diffuse lesion configuration

Exam

- Iris melanoma
  - Heterochromia, corectopia, secondary glaucoma, hyphema, angle seeding, ectropion uveae
  - Dysplastic nevus

    Increased risk of malignant transformation if: age <40 years, hyphema, inferior location of lesion, diffuse/flat configuration, indistinct margins or ectropion uveae
- Posterior uveal melanoma
  - Dome- or mushroom-shaped mass, retinal detachment, pigmented lesion, overlying hemorrhage
  - Dysplastic choroidal/ciliary body nevus

    Increased risk of malignant transformation if: >2 mm thick, acoustically hollow on ultrasound, peripapillary location, orange color, symptomatic, presence of subretinal fluid or absence of drusen/halo sign

Imaging

- Ultrasonography
  - Amplitude scan (A-scan): Medium-to-low reflectivity
  - Brightness scan (B-scan): Hypo-echogenic (acoustically hollow) mass with high height-to-base ratio; "mushroom"
- Fluorescein angiography
  - Persistent early and late hyperfluorescence, "double circulation" pattern if Bruch's membrane is ruptured
- Computed tomography (CT): Hyperdense lesion with moderate contrast enhancement
- Magnetic resonance imaging (MRI): T1 hyperintense and T2 hypointense

Differential Diagnosis

- *Iris melanoma*
  - If lesion is well-circumscribed: iris nevus, iris cyst, sarcoidosis, juvenile xanthogranuloma, leiomyoma, ocular metastasis, ocular melanocytosis
  - If lesion is diffuse: iridocorneal endothelial (ICE) syndrome, congenital heterochromia, ectropion iridis, siderosis, pigmentary glaucoma
- *Posterior uveal melanoma*
  - Choroidal nevus
  - Congenital hypertrophy of the retinal pigment epithelium
  - Choroidal hemangioma
  - Retinal detachment
  - Age-related macular degeneration
  - Peripheral exudative hemorrhagic chorioretinopathy

Treatment

- *Iris melanoma*
  - Monitor with serial photography if the lesion is <3 mm in diameter
  - If growth is noted or the lesion is >3 mm in diameter
    Partial iridectomy
    Iridotrabeculectomy (if anterior chamber angle is involved)
    Iridocyclectomy (if ciliary body is involved)
  - If not resectable: plaque radiotherapy or enucleation (if visual prognosis is poor)
- *Posterior uveal melanoma*
  - Treatment is indicated if at least two risk factors are present (See above under Epidemiology and Prognosis)
  - Plaque radiotherapy with or without transpupillary thermoplasty
  - Photodynamic therapy (for amelanotic lesions)
  - External beam radiotherapy
  - Enucleation, orbital exenteration

66 Benign Lymphoid Hyperplasia of the Uvea

Overview

- A benign, idiopathic lymphoplasmacytic infiltration of the uvea
  - Lymphomatous transformation exceedingly rare
  - Good visual prognosis
  - Rare associations with Castleman's disease and Waldenstrom macroglobulinemia
- Unilateral presentation, typically in adults

Exam

- Conjunctival salmon patch
- Multiple yellow-orange choroidal lesions
- Clear vitreous

Imaging

- Ultrasonography
  - Diffuse choroidal thickening with or without an ovoid echolucent epibulbar mass
- Fluorescein and indocyanine green angiography
  - Early hypofluorescent choroidal lesions with late mild hyperfluorescence

C. S. Foster et al. (eds.), *Uveitis*, https://doi.org/10.1007/978-3-030-52974-1_66

Laboratory and Radiographic Studies

- Rule out systemic and/or central nervous system lymphoma
- Fine needle aspiration of conjunctival lesion or uvea
  - Analysis with immunohistochemistry, polymerase chain reaction, and/or flow cytometry

Differential Diagnosis

- Intraocular lymphoma
- Birdshot retinochoroiditis
- Sarcoidosis
- Amelanotic choroidal melanoma

Treatment

- Oral or periocular steroids
- Ocular irradiation in refractory cases

Juvenile Xanthogranuloma

67

Overview

- Definition
  - A benign non-Langerhans cell histiocytosis of childhood
  - Presents with reddish-yellow cutaneous and iris lesions with spontaneous hyphema that can lead to secondary glaucoma
- Symptoms
  - Typically asymptomatic, but patient may present with blurry vision or red eye
  - Cutaneous lesions are asymptomatic
- Laterality
  - Unilateral
- Course
  - Cutaneous lesions regress within 5 years
- Age of onset
  - Infants and young children
  - Adult variants are known to exist, and lesions are less likely to spontaneously regress
- Gender/race
  - Unknown
- Systemic association
  - Skin: typically a single reddish-yellow papule

C. S. Foster et al. (eds.), *Uveitis*, https://doi.org/10.1007/978-3-030-52974-1_67

Exam: Ocular

Anterior

- Heterochromia iridis
- Spontaneous hyphema
- Yellowish-tan, vascularized, elevated iris lesion

Posterior

- None

Exam: Systemic

- Cutaneous reddish-yellow papules
  - Spontaneously regress within 5 years

Imaging

- Anterior segment OCT
  - Thin, flat, iridic mass

Laboratory and Radiographic Testing

- Fine needle aspiration
  - Touton giant cells
  - Large histiocytes with foamy cytoplasm and scattered eosinophils

Differential Diagnosis

- Neoplasia
  - Retinoblastoma
  - Leukemic infiltrates
- Retinopathy of prematurity
- Sarcoidosis
- Sickle cell anemia

Treatment

Treatment of iris lesions is aimed to prevent the development of secondary glaucoma

- Topical, oral, or periocular steroids
  - Typically a good response
- Resection of iris lesion
  - For recalcitrant lesions

Referral/Co-management

- Dermatology

Retinitis Pigmentosa

68

Overview

- Definition
  - A heterogeneous group of inherited retinal dystrophies primarily affecting the rod photoreceptors, with progressive involvement of the cone photoreceptors and retinal pigment epithelium
    - The most common form of inherited blindness
- Symptoms
  - Nyctalopia
  - Ring scotoma
    - Typically with superior field affected first
    - Symmetric involvement (except in X-linked female carriers)
    - Slow and relentless progression
  - Metamorphopsia (from macular edema)
  - Late stage: dyschromatopsia and vision loss
- Laterality
  - Bilateral
- Course
  - Slow and relentless progression
- Age of onset
  - First to second decade of life
- Gender/race
  - Not applicable
- Systemic association
  - Sensorineural hearing loss (30% of patients with retinitis pigmentosa [RP])
  - A variety of syndromes are associated with RP:
    - Usher syndrome, Bardet-Biedl syndrome, Senior Loken syndrome, adult Refsum disease, etc.

C. S. Foster et al. (eds.), *Uveitis*, https://doi.org/10.1007/978-3-030-52974-1_68

Exam: Ocular

Anterior Segment

- Posterior subcapsular cataract

Posterior Segment

- Bone spicules
- Waxy optic disc pallor
- Arteriolar attenuation
- Cystoid macular edema
- Disc drusen
- Vitreous cells

Exam: Systemic

- Hearing loss

Imaging

- OCT
  - CME
  - Outer retinal atrophy
- ERG
  - Flat or "extinguished"
- Humphrey visual field (static automated perimetry) (HVF)
  - Ring scotoma, most notable on Goldmann kinetic perimetry
- Fundus autofluorescence
  - Perifoveal hyperautofluorescent ring with midperipheral hypoautofluorescent spicules

Laboratory and Radiographic Testing

- Genetic testing
  - Autosomal dominant RP: mild course with variable penetrance; mutations in rhodopsin and peripherin/RDS genes
  - Autosomal recessive RP: severe course with early onset
  - X-linked RP: very severe course with mutations in RPGR gene

Differential Diagnosis

- Autoimmune retinopathy
- Drug-induced retinal toxicity (e.g., thioridazine, chlorpromazine, chloroquine, hydroxychloroquine)
- Pigmented paravenous retinochoroidal atrophy (PPRCA)
- Rubella retinitis
- Traumatic retinopathy
- Syndromic pigmentary retinopathy
  - Including: Bardet-Biedl syndrome, Usher syndrome, Leber's congenital amaurosis, neuronal ceroid lipofuscinosis, Kearns-Sayre syndrome, Batten disease, Refsum disease, abetalipoproteinemia, and Senior Loken syndrome.
- Congenital stationary night blindness (CSNB)
- Choroideremia
- Stargardt maculopathy
- Bietti crystalline dystrophy
- Vitamin A or zinc deficiency
- Syphilis
- Diffuse unilateral subacute neuroretinitis (DUSN)

Treatment

- Referral to low vision specialist
- Limitation of ultraviolet (UV) light exposure
- Cataract extraction
- For CME: topical or oral carbonic anhydrase inhibitors; intravitreal triamcinolone
- Dietary modification:
  - Vitamin A 15,000 IU daily
  - ± docosahexaenoic acid (DHA) 1200 mg daily
  - ± lutein 12–20 mg daily

Referral/Co-management

- Low vision specialist
- Genetic counseling

Intraocular Foreign Body

69

Overview

- Definition
  - Foreign body within the eye introduced by penetrating trauma or surgery
- Symptoms
  - Recent or remote trauma, particularly metal-on-metal work
  - Pain, redness, photophobia, blurry vision
- Laterality
  - Unilateral
- Course
  - Copper is particularly inflammatory; other materials resolve more quickly
- Age of onset
  - All are susceptible, but age 20–40 years most common
- Gender/race
  - More commonly males
- Systemic association
  - None

Exam: Ocular

Anterior

- Cells and flare
- Hypopyon
- Iris transillumination defect
- Corneal wound

C. S. Foster et al. (eds.), *Uveitis*, https://doi.org/10.1007/978-3-030-52974-1_69

Posterior

- Foreign body
- Vitreous hemorrhage
- Traumatic chorioretinopathy

Exam: Systemic

- n/a

Imaging

- Ultrasonography
- Anterior segment Ocular coherence tomography (OCT)
  - Look for intraocular foreign body (IOFB) in the angle structures

Laboratory and Radiographic Testing

- Computed tomography (CT)
  - First-line choice is thin-slice (<1 mm) sections through the globe and orbit.
  - Wood is hypointense; metal is hyperintense.
- Magnetic resonance imaging (MRI)
  - If CT scan has ruled out a metallic foreign body, then MRI is useful for precise localization or detection of wooden foreign bodies.

Differential Diagnosis

- Panuveitis (autoimmune)
- Endophthalmitis

Treatment

- Hospitalization, nil per os (NPO) (i.e. nothing by mouth), and rigid shield over affected eye
- Tetanus prophylaxis
- Broad-spectrum intravenous antibiotics
- Surgical removal of IOFB
- Long-term follow-up with electroretinograms (ERGs) to assess for occult retinal toxicity

Referral/Co-management

- None

Drug-Induced Uveitis

70

Overview

- A thorough review of medications should be conducted in evaluation of every uveitis patient
- Mechanisms of drug-induced uveitis are poorly understood, but may include direct medication toxicity, breakdown of blood-aqueous and blood-retina barriers, and immune-mediated vasculitis
- Using the 10 criteria proposed by Naranjo et al., the causative relationship between a medication and an adverse reaction can be quantitatively assessed

Systemic Medications

Bisphosphonate

- A group of medications used to treat osteoporosis or to prevent fractures in bone malignancy
- Conjunctivitis, anterior uveitis, episcleritis, and scleritis may occur within 24 hours of administration
- Mechanism: release of inflammatory cytokines

Cidofovir

- Given intravenously or intraocularly for CMV retinitis; rarely used today due to irreversible nephrotoxicity
- Nongranulomatous anterior uveitis and hypotony, especially after multiple intraocular injections

C. S. Foster et al. (eds.), *Uveitis*, https://doi.org/10.1007/978-3-030-52974-1_70

- May require aggressive topical or periocular steroids, cycloplegia, and discontinuation of cidofovir; oral probenecid reduces incidence of uveitis and hypotony

Rifabutin

- Used for *Mycobacterium avium* complex prophylaxis in immunocompromised patients
- Characteristic hypopyon anterior uveitis, though intermediate uveitis with dense vitritis, panuveitis, and retinal vasculitis can occur as well
- Incidence is dose and duration dependent (5.6% incidence with 300 mg daily dose, but quadruples with 600 mg)
- Uveitis may be accompanied by arthralgia, jaundice, pseudojaundice, or transient rash
- Uveitis resolves after 1–2 months with intensive topical or systemic corticosteroids and discontinuation of rifabutin

Sulfonamides "Sulfa Drugs"

- Trimethoprim-sulfamethoxazole (Bactrim): bilateral nongranulomatous anterior uveitis. Retinal hemorrhages may appear within a week of taking medication. The trimethoprim component, a non-sulfa drug, can lead to uveitis as well
- Topiramate (Topamax): bilateral anterior uveitis with, uveal effusion. Secondary angle closure may classically result from the effusion displacing the lens/iris diaphragm forward, and anterior rotation of ciliary body

TNF-Alpha Inhibitors

- Etanercept (Enbrel), infliximab (Remicade), and adalimumab (Humira) have all been implicated – particularly etanercept – in paradoxical autoimmune reactions, including uveitis, biopsy-proven sarcoidosis (as well as ocular sarcoidosis), lupus-like syndrome, interstitial lung disease, and autoimmune hepatitis
- Most reported cases occur within 1 year of therapy start and most resolve after discontinuation of TNF-alpha inhibitors
- Mechanism: auto-antibody formation and subsequent immune complex deposition

Fluoroquinolones

- Acute, bilateral anterior uveitis, often within 3–4 weeks of exposure. May have significant pigment dispersion, endothelial dusting, iris atrophy, posterior synechiae, and possible IOP elevation
- Iris transillumination defect and mydriasis may persist after acute episode

Immune Checkpoint Inhibitors (ICPIs): Ipilimumab, Pembrolizumab, Nivolumab

- Tumor cells evade the immune system by activating inhibitory receptors, including CTLA-4 and PD-1, on the surface of tumor-specific T lymphocytes
- Ipilimumab (Yervoy) binds CTLA-4, while Pembrolizumab (Keytruda) and Nivolumab (Opdivo) bind PD-1 to prevent such inactivation by tumor cells:
  - Ipilimumab indicated for metastatic cutaneous melanoma
  - Pembrolizumab and nivolumab indicated for a variety of malignancies in addition to melanoma
- All 3 ICIPs have been associated with bilateral uveitis, most commonly anterior but also intermediate, posterior and panuveitis. Posterior segment presentation can be highly VKH-like
- Typical onset: 6–12 weeks after ICPI infusion
- Uveitis accounts for about 1% of all adverse events associated with ICPIs, while colitis accounts for up to 60%. Other systemic manifestations include vitiligo, hearing loss, poliosis, headache, arthritis, rash, autoimmune hepatitis, interstitial nephritis, pneumonitis
- Topical, regional, or systemic corticosteroid may need to be maintained if ICPI needs to be continued
- Mechanisms: T-cell activation and, in cases of cutaneous and choroidal melanomas, tumor lysis result in melanin and melanin-associated protein release into bloodstream, which in turn activate primed T-cells in the uveal tract

BRAF Inhibitors (Vemurafenib, Dabrafenib) and MEK Inhibitors (Trametinib)

- Inhibit signaling pathways that lead to tumor proliferation
- Indicated for metastatic cutaneous melanoma
- All 3 have been associated with bilateral uveitis, most commonly anterior

Topical Medications

Brimonidine

- Granulomatous anterior uveitis with IOP elevation, conjunctival hyperemia, and follicular conjunctivitis
- Usually occurs after 1+ year of use
- When used bilaterally, uveitis onset in each eye can be asynchronous, with a long delay in fellow eye involvement
- Mechanism: unknown

Metipranolol

- Granulomatous anterior uveitis
- Mechanism: unknown

Prostaglandin Analogues

- Latanoprost, travoprost, and bimatoprost have all been associated with anterior uveitis, with latanoprost most frequently implicated
- Mechanisms: breakdown of blood-aqueous barrier, increased production of inflammatory mediators such as IL-1, IL-6, and eicosanoids
- Other side effects of prostaglandin analogues: conjunctival hyperemia, eyelash growth, iris darkening, periocular skin pigmentation, CME, and reactivation of HSV keratitis
- We find this class of glaucoma drops to have effective IOP-reducing effect and do not lead to increased flare-ups in our uveitis patients, as long as disease is controlled with systemic IMT

Intraocular Medications

Anti-VEGF

- Acute intraocular inflammation with severe complications has been reported especially with bevacizumab
- Symptoms of decreased vision and floaters that often start within 24 hours of injection
- Patients respond to systemic or topical corticosteroid treatment with a slow but persistent recovery
- Pain may be the only symptom that distinguishes true infectious endophthalmitis from a sterile intraocular inflammation secondary to anti-VEGF

Triamcinolone Acetonide

- Sterile endophthalmitis similar to that seen with anti-VEGF
- Likely due to preservatives, as introduction of preservative-free formulation (Triesence) has greatly reduced incidence

Vaccines

Most cases presented with anterior chamber reaction and mild papillitis, resolved with topical steroids or observation only

- BCG (definite)
- Influenza (probable)
- MMR (probable)
- Hepatitis B (probable)
- HPV (probable)
- Varicella (possible)

Drug-Induced TINU Syndrome

All are single-case reports, presented with acute interstitial nephritis on renal biopsy but developed bilateral anterior uveitis 1–3 months after drug discontinuation

- Flubiprofen
- *Goreisan* (a Chinese herb)
- Paracetamol
- Codeine phosphate
- Lamotrigine
- Smoking synthetic cannabinoid

Uveitis During Pregnancy

71

Overview

- Noninfectious uveitis in pregnancy shows increased disease activity early in pregnancy, significant reduction in activity in late trimesters, and rebound inflammation postpartum
- Infectious uveitis, especially toxoplasma retinochoroiditis, may have a higher incidence of reactivation during pregnancy
- When considering treatment, the risks and benefits to the fetus and mother must always be carefully weighed, with knowledge that severe, untreated inflammatory disease in the mother is possibly harmful to the fetus

Clinical Course

- Hormonal changes in pregnancy ultimately decrease cell-mediated inflammation by upregulating Th2 cells and downregulating Th1 cells
  - These changes are driven by increased levels of estrogen, progesterone, alpha fetoprotein, cortisol, norepinephrine, prolactin, and 1,25-dihydroxyvitamin D
- Improved disease activity in patients with Adamantiades-Behcet's disease, VKH syndrome, sympathetic ophthalmia, HLA-B27 associated anterior uveitis, rheumatoid arthritis, juvenile idiopathic arthritis (JIA), and multiple sclerosis
  - There is notable inflammatory rebound in the 6 months after parturition
- Potential worsening of systemic lupus erythematosus (SLE) disease activity
- Rates of *de novo* infection and reactivation of toxoplasma retinochoroiditis are increased

C. S. Foster et al. (eds.), *Uveitis*, https://doi.org/10.1007/978-3-030-52974-1_71

- Considerations for immunosuppression:
  - Although IMT carries risks, it is likely that untreated, severe disease also poses harm to the fetus
  - Non-infectious uveitis in pregnancy:
    Prednisone and prednisolone (FDA Pregnancy Category B) are safe during pregnancy and breastfeeding
    - Dose exceeding 9 mg/day may be associated with fetal cleft palate and a theoretical risk of premature rupture of membranes or chorioamnionitis

    Azathioprine (Category D) may be safely continued in pregnant women with severe disease at doses ≤2 mg/kg/day
    Methotrexate, mycophenolate mofetil, and alkylating agents (Category X) are known teratogens and must be avoided in pregnancy and discontinued at least 3 months prior to conception
    Tacrolimus and cyclosporine (Category C) are safe in low doses but should be avoided during breastfeeding
    TNF-α inhibitors (Category B) appear to be safe and well-tolerated in pregnancy
    Tocilizumab (Category C) and its effect on pregnancy have not been studied in humans
    Rituximab (Category C) may cause neonatal B-cell lymphocytopenia and should be discontinued 1 year prior to conception
  - Infectious uveitis in pregnancy:
    Toxoplasma retinochoroiditis:
    - Spiramycin 1 g TID is drug of choice during early pregnancy (<18 weeks gestation)
      - Significantly lowers vertical transmission rate
      - Licensed in Canada and Europe but available in the USA only directly through the FDA
    - Trimethoprim/sulfamethoxazole 160/800 mg BID can be used in late second or third trimester

    Syphilitic uveitis:
    - Intravenous penicillin 18–24 million units/day for 2 weeks

Correction to: Uveitis

C. Stephen Foster, Stephen D. Anesi, and Peter Y. Chang

Correction to: C. S. Foster et al. (eds.), Uveitis, https://doi.org/10.1007/978-3-030-52974-1

The book was inadvertently published with incorrect authorships in Chapter 27, and 31. It has been updated as follows:

Chapter 27
From "Koushik Tripathy, Aniruddha Agarwal" to "Koushik Tripathy, Aniruddha Agarwal, and Miriam Baron Barshak".

Chapter 31
"Jordan A. Ueberroth" to "Jordan A. Ueberroth and Miriam Baron Barshak".

The updated versions of the chapters can be found at
https://doi.org/10.1007/978-3-030-52974-1_27
https://doi.org/10.1007/978-3-030-52974-1_31

C. S. Foster et al. (eds.), *Uveitis*, https://doi.org/10.1007/978-3-030-52974-1_72

Appendix I: SUN Nomenclature

Table A.1 SUN Working Group anatomical classification of uveitis

Type	Primary site of inflammation	Includes
Anterior	Anterior chamber	Iritis
		Iridocyclitis
		Anterior cyclitis
Intermediate	Vitreous	Pars planitis
		Posterior cyclitis
		Hyalitis
Posterior	Retina or choroid	Focal, multifocal or diffuse choroiditis
		Chorioretinitis
		Retinochoroiditis
		Retinitis
		Neuroretinitis
Panuveitis	Anterior chamber, vitreous, and retina or choroid	

Adapted from Jabs DA, Nussenblatt RB, Rosenbaum JT. Standardization of Uveitis Nomenclature (SUN) Working Group. Standardization of uveitis nomenclature for reporting clinical data. Results of the First International Workshop. *Am J Ophthalmol.* 2005;140(3): 509–16

Table A.2 SUN Working Group grading scheme for anterior chamber cells

Grade	Cells in field[a]
0	<1
0.5+	1–5
1+	6–15
2+	16–25
3+	26–50
4+	>50

Adapted from Jabs DA, Nussenblatt RB, Rosenbaum JT. Standardization of Uveitis Nomenclature (SUN) Working Group. Standardization of uveitis nomenclature for reporting clinical data. Results of the First International Workshop. *Am J Ophthalmol.* 2005;140(3): 509–16
[a]Field size is a 1 mm by 1 mm slit beam

C. S. Foster et al. (eds.), *Uveitis*, https://doi.org/10.1007/978-3-030-52974-1

Table A.3 SUN Working Group grading scheme for anterior chamber flare

Grade	Description
0	None
1+	Faint
2+	Moderate (iris and lens details clear)
3+	Marked (iris and lens details hazy)
4+	Intense (fibrin or plastic aqueous)

Adapted from Jabs DA, Nussenblatt RB, Rosenbaum JT. Standardization of Uveitis Nomenclature (SUN) Working Group. Standardization of uveitis nomenclature for reporting clinical data. Results of the First International Workshop. *Am J Ophthalmol*. 2005;140(3): 509–16

Table A.4 SUN Working Group descriptors in uveitis

Category	Descriptor	Comment
Onset	Sudden	
	Insidious	
Duration	Limited	≤3 Months duration
	Persistent	≥3 Months duration
Course	Acute	Episode of sudden onset and limited duration
	Recurrent	Repeat episodes separated by periods of inactivity without therapy ≥3 months duration
	Chronic	Persistent with relapse in <3 months after discontinuing therapy

Adapted from Jabs DA, Nussenblatt RB, Rosenbaum JT. Standardization of Uveitis Nomenclature (SUN) Working Group. Standardization of uveitis nomenclature for reporting clinical data. Results of the First International Workshop. *Am J Ophthalmol*. 2005;140(3): 509–16

Table A.5 SUN Working Group Activity of uveitis terminology

Term	Definition
Inactive	Grade 0 cells (in anterior chamber)
Worsening activity	2-Step *increase* in level of inflammation (i.e., anterior chamber cells, vitreous haze) or *increase* from grade 3+ to 4+
Improved activity	2-Step *decrease* in level of inflammation (i.e., anterior chamber cells, vitreous haze) or *decrease* to grade 0
Remission	Inactive disease for ≥3 months after discontinuing all therapy for eye disease

Adapted from Jabs DA, Nussenblatt RB, Rosenbaum JT. Standardization of Uveitis Nomenclature (SUN) Working Group. Standardization of uveitis nomenclature for reporting clinical data. Results of the First International Workshop. *Am J Ophthalmol*. 2005;140(3): 509–16

Table A.6 Criteria for grading vitreous flare

Grade	Descriptors
0	No inflammation present
0.5+	Trace inflammation present (slight blurring of optic nerve margins, normal striations, and reflex of nerve fiber layer cannot be visualized)
1+	Mild blurring of the optic nerve and retinal vessels
2+	Optic nerve visible, borders blurred markedly
3+	Optic nerve head not visible
4+	

Adapted from Jabs DA, Nussenblatt RB, Rosenbaum JT. Standardization of Uveitis Nomenclature (SUN) Working Group. Standardization of uveitis nomenclature for reporting clinical data. Results of the First International Workshop. *Am J Ophthalmol*. 2005;140(3): 509–16

Table A.7 Criteria for grading vitreous cells

Grade	Number of vitreous cells
0	No cells
0.5+	1–10
1+	11–20
2+	21–30
3+	31–100
4+	>101

Adapted from Jabs DA, Nussenblatt RB, Rosenbaum JT. Standardization of Uveitis Nomenclature (SUN) Working Group. Standardization of uveitis nomenclature for reporting clinical data. Results of the First International Workshop. *Am J Ophthalmol*. 2005;140(3): 509–16

Appendix II: Pharmacopeia

Table A.8 Systemic medications

Generic name (trade name)	Initial dose (route)	Maximum dose (route)	Mechanism
Cyclophosphamide (Cytoxan)	1 mg/kg/day (PO) or 1 g/m^2 (BSA) infusions q1–2 weeks (IV – pulse)	3 mg/kg/day (PO)	Alkylating agent (DNA crosslinking)
Chlorambucil (Leukeran)	0.15 mg/kg/day (PO)	18 mg/kg/day (PO)	Alkylating agent (DNA crosslinking)

Representative side effects	Lab test – baseline	Lab test – follow up	Comments
Sterile hemorrhagic cystitis (acrolein induced), myelosuppression, reversible alopecia, infections, sterility, secondary malignancies, *blurring of vision, elevated IOP*	CBC and Diff, LFTs, BUN/Cr, UA	CBC and Diff q2 wks, LFTs, BUN/Cr, UA qmnth	The dose for IV infusions is titrated based upon changes in the total WBC count (aim 3500–4500 cells/μL). ANC >1,500 cells/μL, platelet counts >75,000/μL. Cascading trends of counts looked for at every infusion visit. Cryopreservation of sperms and eggs prior to induction PRN. Consumption of 2–4 liters of water daily. Malignancy associated with 76 g (cumulative dose) or 50 mg (daily dose) for more than 2 years.
Reversible myelosuppression (moderate, rapid, protracted), irreversible bone marrow aplasia, gonadal dysfunction, sterility, infections, secondary malignancies	CBC and Diff, LFTs	CBC and Diff q1–3 wks, LFTs q3–4 months	Routine prophylaxis of *Pneumocystis pneumonia* is advised in conjunction.

(continued)

C. S. Foster et al. (eds.), *Uveitis*, https://doi.org/10.1007/978-3-030-52974-1

Table A.8 (continued)

Generic name (trade name)	Initial dose (route)	Maximum dose (route)	Mechanism
Methotrexate (Folex, Mexate, Rheumatrex, Otrexup, Rasuvo)	7.5–15 mg/wk or 0.15 mg/kg/wk (Oral/SC)	20 mg/wk (PO), 50 mg/wk (SC) 200 mg/wk (IV)	Inhibitor of dihydrofolate reductase
Azathioprine (Imuran)	1 mg/kg/day (PO – QD/BID)	3 mg/kg/day (PO)	Alters purine metabolism
Mycophenolate mofetil (Cellcept), Mycophenolate sodium (Myfortic)	1 g (PO – divided dose), Sodium – 360 mg	3 g (PO – divided dose) Sodium – 760 mg (PO), on an empty stomach	Inosine monophosphate dehydrogenase inhibitor (purine synthesis)
Leflunomide (Arava)	100 mg QD × 3 then 20 mg QD or 0.01 mg/kg (PO)	10 mg/kg/day or 20 mg QD (PO)	Inhibits dihydro-orotate dehydrogenase (pyrimidine synthesis)

Representative side effects	Lab test – baseline	Lab test – follow up	Comments
Ulcerative stomatitis, myelosuppression (leukopenia, thrombocytopenia), GI distress, hepatotoxicity (hepatitis, cirrhosis), pulmonary toxicity, cutaneous vasculitis, fetal loss	CBC and Diff, LFTs BUN/Cr, UA	CBC and Diff q1–4 wks, LFTs, BUN/Cr, UA q3–6 wks	Alcoholism and outdoor activity to be avoided. Authors prefer administering doses of above 20 mg/wk by SC mode of administration. IV rescue doses are used sparingly. Administered along with folic acid or leucovorin.
Myelosuppression (leukopenia, thrombocytopenia), GI distress, hepatitis, infections, pancreatitis	CBC and Diff, LFTs, BUN/Cr, TPMT activity	CBC and Diff-q1–4 wks, LFTs, BUN/Cr q3–6 wks	Check TPMT activity: avoid if absent or low.
GI distress, neutropenia, infection	CBC and Diff, LFTs, BUN/Cr	CBC and Diff q1–4 wks, LFTs, BUN/Cr q3–6 wks	
Diarrhea, neurological effects			

Generic name (trade name)	Initial dose (route)	Maximum dose (route)	Mechanism
Cyclosporine (Sandimmune, Neoral, SangCyA)	2.5–5 mg/kg/day (PO – divided dose)	10 mg/kg/day (PO)	Calcineurin inhibitor
Tacrolimus (Prograf, FK 506)	0.05 mg/kg/day (PO)	0.3 mg/kg/day (PO)	Calcineurin inhibitor
Sirolimus (Rapamune, Rapamycin)	Loading: 6 mg/day (PO), Maintenance: 2 mg/day	6 mg/day (PO)	mTOR pathway inhibitor

Table A.8 (continued)

Representative side effects	Lab test: baseline	Lab test: follow-up	Comments
Nephrotoxicity, HT, hyperuricemia, DM, hypercholesterolemia, neurotoxicity, hirsutism, gum hyperplasia	CBC and Diff, BUN/Cr, Cr clearance, LFTs, fasting lipid profile and BP, trough level monitoring	CBC and Diff, BUN/Cr, LFTs, trough level monitoring, BP q1–3 weeks. Fasting lipid profile, Cr clearance q3mnth	Neoral has a greater bioavailability than Sandimmune, so its dose should be reduced by 20% when substituting the drug. Drug and food interactions.
Nephrotoxicity, HT, DM, neurotoxicity	Similar to cyclosporine	Similar to cyclosporine	Can be used in cyclosporine-resistant ocular inflammatory disorders. Drug and food interactions.
GI distress and dermatological manifestations, unknown	Similar to cyclosporine, quantitative urinary protein excretion monitoring	Similar to tacrolimus, periodic quantitative urinary protein excretion monitoring	

Generic name (trade name)	Initial dose (route)	Maximum dose (route)	Mechanism
Adalimumab (Humira)	40 mg every other week after loading (SC)	40 mg qwk (SC)	Fully humanized Ig1 monoclonal anti-TNFα antibody
Infliximab (Remicade)	5–10 mg/kg (IV) q4wk after 2 loading doses in the 1st month (IV)	20 mg/kg (IV)	Chimeric IgG1κ anti-TNFα monoclonal antibody with a human constant & mouse variable region
Abatacept (Orencia)	500–1000 mg q4wk after 3 loading doses in the 1st month (IV) 125 mg qwk (SC)	1000 mg q4wk (IV) 125 mg qwk (SC)	Recombinant soluble fusion protein consists of extracellular domain of human CTLA-4 linked to modified Fc portion of human IgG1.
Certolizumab (Cimzia)	200 mg q2wk or 400 mg q4wk (SC)	400 mg q2wk (SC)	Recombinant human anti-TNFα antibody Fab′ fragment.
Anakinra (Kineret)	100 mg/day (SC)	100 mg/day (SC)	Humanized anti IL-1 receptor monoclonal IgG antibody.
Rituximab (Rituxan)	375 mg/m^2 qwk × 8 then qmnth (IV)	500 mg/m^2 (IV)	Genetically engineered chimeric IgG1κ murine/human anti-CD20 monoclonal antibody.
Golimumab (Simponi)	50–100 mg qmnth after loading (SC)	100 mg qmnth (SC)	Human IgGκ anti-TNF-α monoclonal antibody.
Tocilizumab (INN, Atlizumab, Actemra, Roactemra)	4 mg/kg (IV)	480 mg or 8 mg/kg q4wk (IV)	Recombinant humanized IgG1κ anti IL-6 receptor monoclonal antibody.

(continued)

Table A.8 (continued)

Representative side effects	Lab test: baseline	Lab test – follow-up	Comments
Infections, injection site reactions, headache, rash, demyelinating disease, nonmelanoma skin cancers, TB and Hep B reactivation, drug-induced lupus less likely than with infliximab	CBC and Diff, LFTs, tuberculin testing, Hep B (if at risk)	CBC and Diff, LFTs qvisit, tuberculin testing q1yr, Hep B (if at risk) several months following therapy	Appears safe during pregnancy
Infections, infusion reaction, headache, rash, demyelinating disease, TB and Hep B reactivation, drug-induced lupus	CBC and Diff, LFTs, ANA, tuberculin testing, Hep B (if at risk)	CBC and Diff, LFTs qprior to each infusion, ANA q3mnth; tuberculin testing, Hep B (if at risk) q1yr	"Remicade reaction": Flushing, lower back pain, chest tightness, tachycardia. Concomitant administration with methotrexate to decrease formation of human antichimeric antibodies
Infections, infusion, or injection site reaction, COPD exacerbation, headache, GI upset	CBC and Diff, LFTs	CBC and Diff, LFTs prior to each infusion	
Infections, psoriatic form rashes, TB reactivation	CBC and Diff, LFTs, tuberculin testing, Hep B (if at risk)	CBC and Diff, LFTs prior to each infusion	Appears safe during pregnancy and breastfeeding.
Infections, injection site reaction, rash, GI upset, arthralgia, myalgia	CBC and Diff, LFTs	CBC and Diff, LFTs	
IgE-mediated hypersensitivity to murine proteins, 135, nephrotoxicity, cardiotoxicity	CBC and Diff, CD20+ cells	Prior to each infusion: CBC and Diff, CD20+ cells	
Infections, TB and Hep B reactivation, malignancies, heart failure, demyelinating disease, hypersensitivity reactions	CBC and Diff, LFTs, tuberculin testing, Hep B (if at risk)	CBC and Diff, LFTs	
Infections, gastrointestinal perforation, leucopenia (neutropenia, thrombocytopenia)	CBC and Diff, LFTs, fasting lipid profile, tuberculin testing	CBC and Diff, LFTs prior to each infusion, lipids q4–8wk	At initiation ANC >2000/μL, platelets >1,00,000/μL. Discontinue when ANC <500/μL, platelets <50,000 μL.

Table A.8 (continued)

Generic name (trade name)	Initial dose (route)	Maximum dose (route)	Mechanism
Intravenous immunoglobulin	1–2 g/kg/cycle over 3 days (IV)	2.5 mg/kg split over 3 days (IV)	Intact IgG
Interferon-α 2a (Pegasys, Peginterferon α 2a, Pegintron)	3 million units/day or /3 times a week (SC/IM)	6 million units/ day (SC/IM)	Immunomodulatory cytokine
Interferon-β 1a			Immunomodulatory cytokine

Representative side effects	Lab test: baseline	Lab test: follow-up	Comments
Aseptic meningitis, thromboembolism, risk of transmission of blood-borne infections, CHF			Anti-IgA immunization may occur. Proposed mechanism of action – multiple. OCP – IVIG 1 month prior to Rituximab, then qmnth until B cell levels return to normal. Thereafter, IVIg is administered at 6, 8, 10, 12, 14, and 16 weeks.
Fatal neuropsychiatric, autoimmune, ischemic and infectious disorders	CBC and Diff, LFTs, BUN/Cr		Discontinue if ANC <500/μL, platelets <25,000 μL.
Hepatotoxicity, cardiotoxicity, autoimmune thyroiditis, flu-like symptoms, injection site reactions	CBC and Diff, LFTs, thyroid function tests	CBC, LFTs q4wk, thyroid function tests q3mnth	

Abbreviations: *qwk* Every week, *qmnth* Every month, *qyr* Every year, *qvisit* Every visit, *qprior each infusion* Before every infusion, *QD* Once a day, *BID* Twice a day, *TID* Three times a day, *QID* Four times a day, *GI* Gastrointestinal, *PO* Per oral, *SC* Subcutaneous, *IM* Intramuscular, *IV* Intravenous, *ANC* Absolute neutrophil count, *BUN/Cr* Blood urea nitrogen, serum creatinine, *CBC and Diff* Complete and differential blood count, *LFTs* Liver function tests, *TPMT* Thiopurine S-methyltransferase, *UA* Urine analysis

Table A.9 Mydriatics and cycloplegics

		Mydriasis		Cycloplegia	
Generic name (trade name)	Strength (%)	Maximal (min)	Recovery (days)	Maximal (hour)	Recovery (days)
Atropine sulfate (multiple)	1	30–40	7–10	1–3	7–12
Scopolamine hydrobromide (multiple)	0.5	20–30	3–7	0.5–1	5–7
Homatropine hydrobromide (multiple)	1	40–60	1–3	0.5–1	1–3
Cyclopentolate hydrochloride (multiple)	0.5–1	30–60	1	0.5–1	1
Tropicamide (multiple)	0.5–1	20–40	0.25–1	0.5	<0.25
Phenylephrine hydrochloride (multiple)	0.5–1	20–60	3–6	None	None

Table A.10 Topical corticosteroids

Generic name (trade name)	Formulation
Dexamethasone alcohol (Decadron Phosphate)	0.1% suspension
Dexamethasone sodium phosphate	0.1% solution
Dexamethasone sodium phosphate ointment	0.05% ointment
Prednisolone acetate (Pred Forte, Econopred Plus, AK-Tate)	1.0% suspension
Prednisolone acetate (Pred Mild, Econopred)	0.12% suspension
Prednisolone sodium phosphate (Inflamase Forte, AK-Pred)	1% solution
Prednisolone sodium phosphate (Metreton)	0.5% solution
Prednisolone phosphate (Hydeltrasol)	0.5%, 0.25% ointment
Fluorometholone alcohol (FML)	0.1% or 0.25% suspension
Fluorometholone (FML SOP)	0.1% ointment
Medrysone (HMS)	1% suspension
Rimexolone (Vexol)	1% suspension
Medroxyprogesterone acetate (Provera)	1% suspension
Rimexolone (Vexol)	1.0% suspension
Loteprednol etabonate (Lotemax)	0.5% suspension
Loteprednol etabonate (Alrex)	0.2% suspension
Loteprednol etabonate (Inflamase Mild)	0.12% solution
Difluprednate (Durezol)	0.05% emulsion

Table A.11 Regional corticosteroids

Generic name (trade name)	Dose (route)
Hydrocortisone-100–1000 mg powder (Hydrocortisone Sodium Succinate)	50–125 mg (subconjunctival/ subtenon)
Methylprednisolone sodium succinate-40 mg/ml, 125 mg/ml, 2 g/30 ml solution (Solu-medrol)	40–125 mg (subconjunctival/ subtenon)
Methylprednisolone acetate-20–80 mg/ml (depot) suspension (Depo-medrol)	40–80 mg/0.5 ml (transseptal, retrobulbar)
Triamcinolone diacetate-25–40 mg/ml suspension (Aristocort)	40 mg (subconjunctival/ subtenon)
Triamcinolone acetonide-10–40 mg/ml suspension (Kenalog)	40 mg (transseptal)
Triamcinolone acetonide-40 mg/ml (Triescense)	4 mg (intravitreal)
Dexamethasone acetate-6–16 mg/ml suspension (Decadron-LA)	4–8 mg (subconjunctival/ subtenon/transseptal)
Dexamethasone sodium phosphate-4, 10, 24 mg/ml solution (Decadron Phosphate)	0.4 mg (retrobulbar, intravitreal)
Betamethasone acetate and sodium phosphate-3 mg/ml suspension (Celestone Soluspan)	1 mg (subconjunctival/tenon/ transseptal)

Table A.12 Intravitreal corticosteroid implants

Generic Name (trade name)	Dose	Office procedure	Biodegradable	Maximum effectiveness	Lifespan
Dexamethasone (Ozurdex)	0.7 mg	Yes	Yes	1–3 months	6 months
Fluocinolone acetonide (Yutiq)	0.18 mg	Yes	No		18–36 months
Fluocinolone acetonide (Retisert)	0.59 mg	No	No		18–30 months

Table A.13 Systemic corticosteroids

Generic name (trade name)	Formulation	Duration of action
Hydrocortisone (Cortef)	5–20 mg tablet (PO), 10 mg/5 ml suspension (PO), 25 and 50 mg suspension (IM)	Short
Hydrocortisone (Hydrocortone Phosphate)	50 mg/ml solution (IM/IV)	Short
Hydrocortisone (Solu-Cortef)	100–1000 mg powder (IM/IV)	Short
Prednisone (Deltasone, Meticorten, Drasone)	1–50 mg tablet (PO)	Intermediate
Prednisone (Liquid Pred)	5 mg/ml solution (PO)	Intermediate
Prednisolone (Delta-Cortef)	1–5 mg tablet (PO)	Intermediate
Prednisolone (Prelone)	15 mg/ml syrup (PO)	Intermediate
Prednisolone acetate (Predalone)	25–100 mg/ml suspension (IM)	Intermediate
Prednisolone sodium phosphate (Hydeltrasol)	20 mg/ml solution (IM/IV)	Intermediate
Methylprednisolone (Medrol)	2–32 mg tablet (PO)	Intermediate
Methylprednisolone acetate (Depomedrol)	20–80 mg/ml suspension (IM)	Intermediate
Methylprednisolone sodium succinate (Solumedrol)	40–1000 mg powder (IM/IV)	Intermediate
Triamcinolone diacetate (Kenacort)	4 mg/5 ml (PO)	Intermediate
Triamcinolone diacetate (Aristocort)	1–8 mg tablet (PO), 40 mg/ml suspension (IM)	Intermediate
Triamcinolone acetonide (Kenalog)	10–40 mg/ml suspension (PO)	Long
Dexamethasone sodium (Decadron)	0.25–6 mg tablet (PO), 0.5 mg/5 ml elixir (PO), 0.5 mg/5 ml solution (PO)	Long
Dexamethasone sodium phosphate (Decadron Phosphate)	4–24 mg/ml solution (IM/IV)	Long
Dexamethasone acetate (Decadron-LA)	8 mg/ml suspension	Long
Betamethasone (Celestone)	0.6 mg tablet (PO), 0.6 mg/5 ml syrup (PO)	Long
Betamethasone sodium phosphate (Celestone Phosphate)	3 mg/ml solution (IV)	Long
Betamethasone acetate (Celestone Acetate)	3–6 mg/ml suspension (IM)	Long
Betamethasone acetate and sodium phosphate (Celestone Soluspan)	3 mg/ml suspension each (IM)	Long

Table A.14 Oral NSAIDs

Class of drug	Generic name (trade name)	Dose
Salicylates	Aspirin (Multiple Brands)	650 mg q4hrs
	Diflunisal (Dolobid)	200–500 mg BID
Fenamates	Mefenamat (Ponstel)	250 mg QID
	Meclofenamate (Meclofen)	50–100 mg QID
Indoles	Indomethacin (Indocin)	25–50 mg TID-QID, 75 mg BID
	Sulindac (Clinoril)	150–200 mg BID
	Tolmetin (Tolectin)	400 mg TID

(continued)

Table A.14 (continued)

Class of drug	Generic name (trade name)	Dose
Phenyl acetic acid	Diclofenac (Voltaren)	50–75 mg BID
Phenyl alkanoic acids	Fenoprofen (Nalfon)	300–600 mg TID
	Ketoprofen (Oridus)	75 mg TID-50 mg QID
	Piroxicam (Feldene)	10 mg BID, 20 mg QID
	Flurbiprofen (Ansaid)	100 mg TID
	Ketorolac (Toradol)	10 mg QID
	Naproxen (Naprosyn)	250–500 mg BID
	Naproxen (Anaprox)	275–550 mg BID
	Ibuprofen (Motrin, Brufen, Advil, Nuprin)	400–800 mg TID
Pyrazolons	Phenylbutazone (Butazolidin, Azolid)	100 mg TID-QID
	Oxyphenylbutazone (Tendearil, Osalid)	100 mg TID-QID
Para-aminophenols	Acetaminophen (Multiple)	650 mg q4hrs
Cox-2 inhibitors	Celecoxib (Celebrex)	100–200 mg BID

Index

C. S. Foster et al. (eds.), *Uveitis*, https://doi.org/10.1007/978-3-030-52974-1

MIX
Papier aus verantwortungsvollen Quellen
Paper from responsible sources
FSC® C105338

If you have any concerns about our products,
you can contact us on
ProductSafety@springernature.com

In case Publisher is established outside the EU,
the EU authorized representative is:
Springer Nature Customer Service Center GmbH
Europaplatz 3, 69115 Heidelberg, Germany

Printed by Libri Plureos GmbH
in Hamburg, Germany